CONTENTS

Brackets indicate the number of questions in each subject.

FOREWORD

MEDICINE International, the monthly add-on journal, has been published in the UK since 1972. The worldwide readership of the English language editions of the journal approaches 250,000 copies per month, with a distribution covering 110 countries

Multiple choice questions related to the content of the journal have appeared regularly since the beginning of the first series as an integral part of the journal. In addition, a number of booklets have been published containing further questions relating to the journal. These booklets have been well received because they provide a painless and convenient method for the reader to test his knowledge of the content of the journal and especially, because they closely parallel the kind of questions which appear in so many examinations - especially postgraduate diplomas such as the MRCP, MRCGP and their equivalents around the world.

Over the years, we have made determined efforts to maintain the high quality of the multiple choice questions in the journal. Our collaboration with PasTest has enabled us to produce questions of a consistently high standard. This third book contains a large selection of questions on all aspects of clinical internal medicine.

We hope that readers worldwide will find this book of value.

Margaret Stearn MRCP
Medical Editor
MEDICINE International.

INTRODUCTION

The aim of this book is to help the busy doctor test his medical knowledge in his occasional free moments or, if he is working for examinations, to enable him to revise in a methodical manner.

Systematic use of the book should indicate to the reader the subject areas in which he would benefit from further study.

HOW TO USE THIS BOOK

The book can be used on its own as there are brief explanations of the correct answers to all the questions. You will however, obtain far more benefit from the book if you use it in association with MEDICINE International.

Each question is referenced to a particular issue and international page number in all editions of the most recent articles of MEDICINE International.

These references are to be found in the answer section of this book from page 99 onwards. The information on page vii will enable readers around the world to use the local edition of MEDICINE International for reference.

Your method of use of this book will depend on your educational needs and your personal preference. The questions can, of course, be used before and/ or after reading the appropriate sections in the journal and many readers find it helpful to 'pre-test' themselves before deciding upon necessary reading, subsequently 'post-testing' themselves.

Individual study:

● Do not attempt too many questions at one sitting - in this way you are more likely to retain the new knowledge acquired.

● Limit yourself to one group of questions dealing with a specific topic - this should help you to discover your weak points and enable you to use MEDICINE International to revise them.

● Try to avoid looking at the answers before making a definite decision with supporting arguments.

Group discussions:

This can be an effective way to use the book. Ask all participants to test themselves in advance on a set of self-assessment questions and to study their answers in conjunction with the appropriate issues of MEDICINE International. Then discuss the answers with the other members of the group and make further reference to the journal if necessary.

MEDICINE International: you will get maximum value from these questions if you subscribe to MEDICINE International and read each issue as you receive it. The journal contains additional questions, not published in this book, relating to new material as it is published.

PASTEST: if you are working for examinations, other PasTest publications may be of great value to you. There are revision books and/or practice exams available for those preparing for MRCP I & II, MRCGP, MRCOG, Primary FRCS, FCAnaes and PLAB.

MEDICINE INTERNATIONAL

References to further reading in MEDICINE International second series are given in the answer section of this book.

EXAMINATION TECHNIQUE

The multiple choice questions found in this book are based on the format used in many postgraduate examinations such as the MRCP I, MRCGP, MRCOG, Primary FRCS etc. Each question consists of an initial statement (or 'stem') followed by five possible completions (or 'items') identified by A,B,C,D,E. There is no restriction on the number of true or false items in a question. It is possible for all the items in a question to be true or for all to be false.

The four most important points of technique are:

(1) Read the question carefully and be sure you understand it.
(2) Mark your responses clearly, correctly and accurately.
(3) Use reasoning to work out answers, but if you do not know the answer and cannot work it out, indicate 'Don't Know'.
(4) The best way to obtain a good mark is to have as wide a knowledge as possible of the topics being tested in the examination.

To get the best value from this book you should arrive at an answer either 'True' or 'False' or 'Don't Know' for each item. Commit yourself before you look at the answer - this is really the best way to test your knowledge. In practice you can use the letters 'T', 'F' or 'D' to mark your answer against the question in the book. Alternatively you can prepare a grid on a separate piece of paper thus:-

	A	B	C	D	E
23					
24					

You can then mark your answers on the grid as you go along. To calculate your score give yourself (+1) for each correct item, (-1) for each incorrect item and zero for each 'Don't Know' answer.

All too often examination candidate's marks suffer through an inability to organise their time or through failure to read the instructions carefully. You must ruthlessly allocate your time. For example: in the MRCP Part I there are 60 questions to complete in 2 1/2 hours, that is 2 1/2 minutes per question or 10 questions in 25 minutes. Make sure that you are getting through the exam at this pace or a little quicker to allow time at the end for revision and a re-think on some questions you found difficult.

You must read the question (both stem and items) carefully. You should be quite clear that you know what you are being asked to do. Once you know this, you should indicate your responses by marking the paper boldly, correctly and clearly. In an official examination take great care not to mark the wrong boxes and think very carefully before making a mark on the computer answer sheet. Regard each item as being independent of every other item - each refers to a specific quantum of knowledge. The item (or the stem and the item taken together) make up a statement.

You are required to indicate whether you regard this statement as 'True or 'False' and you are also able to indicate 'Don't Know. Look only at a single statement when answering - disregard all the other statements presented in the question, they have nothing to do with the item you are concentrating on.

Since the answer sheets will be read by a computer they must be filled out in accordance with the instructions. As you go through the questions you can either mark your answers immediately on the answer sheet or mark them in the question book in the first instance, transferring them to the answer sheets at the end. In view of the time pressure you may be best advised to mark your answers on the answer sheets as you go along. Don't worry about marking the answer sheet very neatly the first time. Try to leave time to go over your answers again before the end, in particular going back over any difficult questions which you should have marked clearly in your question book. At the same time you can check that you have marked the answer sheet correctly.

Candidates are frequently uncertain whether or not to guess the answer. Experience shows that you should back your 'hunches'. Only if you are completely in the dark should you record a 'Don't Know' answer. Thus, if the question gives you a clue or your knowledge is sufficient to give you a 'hunch' about the correct answer, you will probably gain from guessing.

The answers and explanations in this book are necessarily brief, but they do provide a useful form of revision. The MEDICINE International references with each question give all the background information required to answer that question correctly.

INFECTIONS AND TROPICAL DISEASES

1. **Active immunisation against measles with live attenuated virus**

    A   is recommended by WHO to be given at 9 months
    B   may be ineffective if the child still has high levels of maternal antibody
    C   can be given in the form of an aerosol
    D   is dangerous to babies with protein-energy malnutrition
    E   is more successful in developing than in developed countries

2. **The following are correct statements regarding malaria prophylaxis:**

    A   Fansidar should not be given in combination with chloroquine
    B   chloroquine is available from chemists without prescription
    C   Fansidar must never be taken during pregnancy
    D   chloroquine is safe in pregnancy
    E   chemoprophylaxis should begin 1 week before entering the malarious area

3. **Something more serious than a minor infection should be suspected as the cause of a fever if the patient**

    A   is less than 10 days old
    B   is a child who also complains of headache
    C   is taking immunosuppressive drugs
    D   has recently returned from a visit to Lagos
    E   is a child with a persistent cough

4. **The following neoplasms have a particular tendency to cause obscure fever:**

    A   Hodgkin's disease
    B   hepatoma
    C   renal haemangiopericytoma
    D   atrial myxoma
    E   cerebellar haemangioblastoma

5. **The immunisation schedule recommended by the DHSS for babies between 3 and 12 months of age is intended to provide protection against**

    A   diphtheria
    B   tetanus
    C   rubella
    D   measles
    E   poliomyelitis

6. **Active immunisation is at present available against**

    A   mumps
    B   pneumococcal infections
    C   rabies
    D   hepatitis A
    E   hepatitis B

7. **The period of incubation is less than seven days for**

    A   diphtheria
    B   mumps
    C   rubella
    D   scarlet fever
    E   malaria

8. **The following features are common to infectious mononucleosis, acquired cytomegalovirus infection and glandular toxoplasmosis:**

    A   a positive Paul-Bunnell test
    B   occurrence of chronic latent infection
    C   risk of fatal outcome in the presence of immune deficiency
    D   occasional infection via blood transfusion
    E   in infections in pregnant women, serious risk to the fetus

9. **In treating the following conditions, the drug mentioned should be the primary agent selected:**

    A   Legionnaire's disease: erythromycin
    B   pseudo-membranous colitis: clindamycin
    C   urinary infection with *Pseudomonas aeruginosa*: mecillinam
    D   osteomyelitis due to *Staphylococcus aureus*: carbenicillin
    E   *Haemophilus influenzae* meningitis: chloramphenicol

10. **In the diagnosis of brucellosis**

    A the standard agglutination test (SAT) is the usual procedure for early diagnosis
    B an SAT titre of over 80 is diagnostic
    C persistently negative SAT tests rule out the diagnosis
    D persistence of specific IgG antibodies points to active infection
    E in acute disease, the titre of IgM antibody is less than that of IgG or IgA

11. **The following drug toxicity reactions are not unexpected:**

    A optic neuritis with ethambutol
    B peripheral neuropathy with metronidazole
    C megaloblastic anaemia with trimethoprim
    D hepatitis with pyrazinamide
    E aplastic anaemia with sulphonamides

12. **Antimicrobial treatment is advisable for**

    A *Salmonella* gastroenteritis
    B *Shigella sonnei* infection
    C typhoid fever
    D giardiasis
    E *Yersinia* infections if severe

13. **The following are correct statements about diphtheria:**

    A infection with the mitis strain of the organism causes mild disease only
    B a child with croup and with membrane on the fauces must be regarded as having diphtheria
    C the most reliable early diagnostic aid is the appearance of the Gram-stained smear from the nose or throat
    D extension of the membrane after treatment has begun is an indication that the dose of antitoxin should be repeated
    E the drug of choice to clear *Corynebacterium diphtheriae* from the throat is erythromycin

14.   In tetanus

A   no obvious injury is seen in up to a quarter of all patients
B   bacteriology gives no help in making the diagnosis
C   spasms are invariably accompanied by trismus
D   autonomic instability can be prevented by the total paralysis regime
E   patients surviving the illness have life-long immunity

15.   In typhoid fever

A   animal reservoirs are of increasing importance in maintaining the infection
B   cell-mediated immunity cannot be conferred by immunisation
C   second attacks do not occur
D   the blood culture is positive during the first week of illness
E   chloramphenicol remains the drug of choice in seriously ill patients

16.   The following points are important in the diagnosis of whooping cough:

A   whooping is often absent in neonates
B   there is usually lymphopenia
C   the ESR is nearly always raised
D   bacteriology is of little help
E   whooping does not develop until the second week of illness

17.   The following animals constitute the principal reservoirs of rabies infection in the areas named:

A   Caribbean: mongooses and vampire bats
B   Arctic: polar bears
C   South America: domestic cattle
D   Europe: domestic dog
E   India: monkeys

18. **Factors increasing the likelihood of paralysis in poliomyelitis include**

    A infant status
    B hypodermic injections
    C fatigue
    D physical exercise
    E tonsillectomy

19. **Infections in immunocompromised patients**

    A are generally caused by unusual organisms
    B cause less marked clinical signs than in normal patients
    C progress particularly rapidly if there is neutropenia
    D caused by cytomegalovirus should be treated with acyclovir
    E caused by *Pneumocystis carinii* should be treated with co-trimoxazole

20. **The following are characteristic of the toxic shock syndrome:**

    A multi-system involvement
    B isolation, often in pure culture, of anaerobic streptococci
    C occurrence predominantly in females
    D hypotension
    E a macular rash followed by desquamation of palms and soles

21. **Anthrax**

    A in developed countries usually takes the cutaneous form
    B has an incubation period of about 14 days
    C in the cutaneous form has a fatality rate, untreated, of about 20%
    D does not involve the regional lymph nodes
    E does not cause the formation of pus in the cutaneous lesion

22. **The following drugs are suitable for the treatment of systemic fungal infections:**

    A flucytosine
    B natamycin
    C nystatin
    D amphotericin B
    E miconazole

23.   Mumps

    A   is a notifiable disease in the UK
    B   occurring in a pregnant woman is not an indication for abortion
    C   meningitis is now very rare
    D   affecting both testes usually causes sterility
    E   orchitis can be relieved symptomatically by oral steroids

24.   Infection with herpes simplex virus type 1 (HSV-1)

    A   is more common in lower socio-economic groups
    B   persists in a latent state in sensory ganglia
    C   causes the development of both humoral and cell-mediated immunity
    D   when primary may be symptomless
    E   does not respond to anti-viral drugs

25.   In African trypanosomiasis

    A   the most important diagnostic information is derived from the clinical examination
    B   whenever the diagnosis is made, a lumbar puncture must be performed
    C   blood films should be examined daily for 12 consecutive days
    D   the drug of choice for early *T. brucei rhodesiense* infection is pentamidine
    E   melarsoprol is essential in the treatment if CNS involvement has occurred

26.   The following are correct statements about leishmaniasis:

    A   mucocutaneous leishmaniasis (espundia) is a benign, self-limiting condition
    B   untreated visceral leishmaniasis is usually fatal
    C   visceral leishmaniasis does not occur in the New World
    D   the leishmanin skin test is negative in active visceral leishmaniasis
    E   the drug of choice for visceral leishmaniasis is pentamidine

27. **Vaccines are available for the prevention of**

A Rift Valley fever
B dengue fever
C Omsk haemorrhagic fever
D Lassa fever
E yellow fever

28. **The following arbovirus infections are transmitted to man by mosquito bites:**

A Japanese encephalitis
B Louping ill
C St. Louis encephalitis
D Murray Valley encephalitis
E Crimean-Congo haemorrhagic fever

29. **In amoebic dysentery**

A men are more often affected than women
B the commonest sites for ulcers are the descending colon and the transverse colon
C massive haemorrhage is an important cause of death in untreated cases
D treatment with emetine compounds should be reserved for severely ill patients
E treatment with metronidazole should normally be given for 5 days

30. **In leptospirosis due to infection with *L. interrogans* of the icterohaemorrhagiae serotype**

A the illness is always biphasic
B jaundice does not appear until the 10th day
C death may be due to gastrointestinal haemorrhage
D uveitis is a late complication
E therapy with penicillin must be started in the first week if it is to be effective

31. In tsutsugamushi disease

A   incidence is largely confined to city dwellers
B   small mammals constitute the reservoir of infection
C   patients with G6PD deficiency have an increased risk of developing renal failure
D   the eschar is usually on an exposed area
E   when the diagnosis is certain, the drug of choice is tetracycline

32. Human giardiasis

A   is acquired through the ingestion of cysts
B   occurs principally in the termperate zones
C   has no clearly defined animal reservoir
D   has an incubation period of about 2 weeks
E   affects children more often than adults

33. Diethylcarbamazine is effective in the treatment of infestation with

A   *Loa loa*
B   *Wuchereria bancrofti*
C   *Brugia malayi*
D   *Onchocerca volvulus*
E   *Mansonella streptocerca*

34. In human toxocariasis

A   eosinophilia occurs only rarely
B   damage to the retina, if it occurs, is usually permanent
C   the ELISA test is highly specific
D   cats are a more important source of infection than dogs
E   diethylcarbamazine is effective as a larvicide

35. In tuberculoid (TT) leprosy

A   the skin lesions contain numerous leprosy bacilli
B   thickening of cutaneous nerves may be palpable
C   the lepromin test is positive
D   enlargement of the ear lobes may develop in untreated cases
E   treatment with more than one drug is advised

36. **Infestation with the following is usually acquired by the oral route:**

A   *Ascaris lumbricoides*
B   *Necator americanus*
C   *Strongyloides stercoralis*
D   *Diphyllobothrium latum*
E   *Trichuris trichiura*

37. **In plague**

A   the site of the bite of the infecting flea is usually marked by a painful ulcer
B   the larger the ulcer the worse the prognosis
C   there is usually a neutrophil leucocytosis
D   the drug of choice is chloramphenicol
E   with early treatment the fatality rate is less than 1%

38. **The following are correct statements regarding hydatid disease:**

A   the definitive host for *Echinococcus granulosus* is the dog
B   human infection is acquired from the intermediate host
C   a normal eosinophil count rules out the diagnosis
D   the commonest site for cysts in man is the lung
E   the Casoni skin test is less reliable than *in vitro* serology

39. **In skeletal tuberculosis**

A   the commonest site is the vertebral column
B   abscess formation is uncommon
C   radiography shows the lesions to be surrounded by densely sclerotic new bone
D   survey of the whole skeleton should be performed
E   conventional drug treatment is effective in uncomplicated cases

40. **In *Schistosoma mansoni* infection**

A   hepatic involvement usually causes abnormality of liver function tests
B   diagnosis depends on the identification of the lateral-spined eggs
C   a nephrotic syndrome indicates the deposition of eggs in the glomeruli
D   with gross splenic enlargement, hypersplenism may develop
E   metriphonate is the drug of choice

9

41. In chronic idiopathic urticaria

A the serum IgE level is usually raised
B the patients show other manifestations of atopy
C the onset is usually abrupt
D investigations do not contribute towards making the diagnosis
E antihistamine drugs are the mainstay of treatment

42. In acquired immunodeficiency syndrome (AIDS)

A the patients usually have hypergammaglobulinaemia
B there is anergy to skin test antigens
C infestation of the gut with cryptosporidia is uniformly fatal
D the central pathological feature is a reduction in the number of T suppressor lymphocytes
E the prognosis for those with Kaposi's sarcoma without infection is better

43. Characteristic findings in an anaphylactic attack include

A hypotension
B vomiting
C flushing
D breathlessness
E frequent ventricular ectopic beats

44. The following are correct statements about immunoglobulins:

A serum IgA is predominantly monomeric
B colostrum is rich in secretory IgA
C IgE is secreted by mast cells
D IgM is largely confined to the bloodstream
E combination of IgG with antigen can activate complement

45. The following are manifestations of immune complex disease:

A glomerulonephritis
B nodule formation in rheumatoid arthritis
C acute anaphylaxis
D systemic lupus erythematosus
E drug-induced thrombocytopenia

46. **Significant association of HLA-DR3 with autoimmune reactions has been reported in**

- A Sjögren's syndrome
- B Addison's disease
- C Graves' disease
- D coeliac disease
- E myasthenia gravis

47. **Systemic corticosteroids are of value in the management of**

- A primary vasomotor rhinitis
- B chronic non-specific rhinitis
- C salicylate-associated nasal polyps
- D allergic rhinitis
- E rhinitis medicamentosa

48. **Initial screening tests for suspected immunodeficiency should include**

- A total white cell count and differential
- B total peripheral blood T and B cell numbers
- C total haemolytic complement (CH50) assay
- D serum immunoglobulin levels
- E saliva IgA level

49. Factors contributing to unreliability of clinical trials include

A regression to the mean
B determination of end-point by a single observer
C placebo effect
D crossover design of trial
E prescriber bias

50. The following are correct statements regarding pharmacokinetics:

A the clinical effect of prednisolone is closely related to its plasma concentration
B haemodialysis is the best method of treating overdosage with amitriptyline
C with first order kinetics, the rate of elimination is directly proportional to the concentration of the drug
D lipid-soluble drugs are absorbed more rapidly than water-soluble ones
E drugs excreted as conjugates are dealt with entirely by the kidneys

51. The following drugs act as inducers of hepatic mono-oxygenase activity:

A carbamazepine
B rifampicin
C cimetidine
D metronidazole
E chlorpromazine

52. In the treatment of airway obstruction

A β_2-agonists are preferable to non-selective β-agonists
B nebulized β-agonist is as effective in acute severe asthma as intravenous β-agonist
C the effect of inhaled salbutamol lasts for 1-2 hours only
D there is no good evidence of tolerance to the bronchodilator action of β-agonists
E steroids increase the sensitivity of airway smooth muscle to β-agonists

53. **Measurement of drug levels is clinically helpful in the case of**

   A digoxin
   B ethosuximide
   C procainamide
   D gentamicin
   E sodium valproate

54. **The following drugs act as agonists:**

   A salbutamol
   B disopyramide
   C labetalol
   D apomorphine
   E clonidine

55. **Factors increasing an individual's susceptibility to adverse drug reactions include**

   A Scandinavian racial origin
   B HLA status
   C atopic constitution
   D male sex
   E advanced age

56. **The following drugs are firmly established as teratogenic in humans:**

   A warfarin
   B tetracyclines
   C vitamin D
   D azathioprine
   E diethylstilboestrol

57. **Calcium antagonist drugs**

   A act by blocking the passage of calcium into the cell
   B have a positive inotropic action
   C are ineffective in angina due to coronary artery spasm
   D should never be used in combination with β-blocking drugs
   E reduce blood pressure in hypertension

58. In the drug treatment of hypertension

    A   the diuretic of first choice is frusemide

    B   patients taking thiazide drugs should be given supplementary potassium chloride

    C   patients aged over 80 years of age with uncomplicated hypertension should not be treated

    D   minoxidil should not be given to female patients

    E   atenolol and metoprolol are suitable drugs for patients who also have airways obstruction

59. In the drug treatment of peptic ulceration

    A   carbonoxolone gives healing rates comparable with those for cimetidine

    B   cimetidine causes inhibition of hepatic mono-oxygenase

    C   bismuth chelate gives healing rates no better than those given by a placebo

    D   the main side effect of sucralfate is diarrhoea

    E   bismuth chelate should not be given to pregnant women

60. Warfarin

    A   is rapidly absorbed after oral administration

    B   acts by blocking the absorption of Vitamin K

    C   should be given as life-long therapy to patients with prosthetic heart valves

    D   should not be given to pregnant women

    E   should not be given to patients with chronic liver disease

61. Advantages conferred by the use of oral contraceptives include

    A   suppression of benign breast disease

    B   reduced incidence of carcinoma of ovary

    C   reduced incidence of gallbladder disease

    D   reduced incidence of carcinoma of endometrium

    E   reduced levels of serum triglyceride

62.   Lithium therapy

   A   is unlikely to be beneficial in a single depressive episode
   B   should not be given to pregnant women
   C   may cause weight gain
   D   has a beneficial effect on psoriasis
   E   should be regulated so as to give serum levels of 0.5 - 1 nmol/l

63.   The following are correct statements about the use of anticonvulsant drugs:

   A   elimination of the drugs is predominantly by hepatic metabolism
   B   ethosuximide is effective in petit mal
   C   a single daily dose of carbamazepine is preferable to several divided doses
   D   for patients in whom phenobarbitone causes intolerable side effects, primidone will be a satisfactory alternative
   E   sodium valproate may cause gum hypertrophy

64.   In the treatment of rheumatic disease the following points should be observed:

   A   salicylate drugs should not be given to patients with bronchial asthma
   B   flufenamic acid should not be given to patients with ulcerative colitis
   C   chloroquine should not be given to patients over the age of 55
   D   imminent adverse side effects of gold may be recognised by monitoring serum gold levels
   E   treatment with penicillamine carries a risk of marrow aplasia

65. **Convulsions are an important feature of severe overdose with**

    A diazepam
    B maprotiline
    C amoxapine
    D lithium
    E amitriptyline

66. **The substance quoted after each poison is an effective antidote:-**

    A arsenic: dimercaprol
    B ethylene glycol: ethanol
    C thallium: thiosulphate
    D iron: penicillamine
    E lead: sodium calcium edetate

67. **In the diagnosis and management of poisoning**

    A the patient's statements about the drug ingested are usually unhelpful
    B measurement of blood levels is essential if the toxic agent is iron
    C if hypotension develops, plasma expansion is dangerous
    D skin bullae are diagnostic of barbiturate intoxication
    E self-poisoning is nearly always an indication of psychiatric illness

68. **Methanol poisoning**

    A is most commonly seen in methylated spirit drinkers
    B commonly causes tachypnoea
    C should be treated by haemodialysis if the blood level is over 500 mg/l
    D causes its toxic effect by being converted to formaldehyde and formate
    E may cause clinically apparent papillitis

69. **The metabolic abnormalities caused by salicylate intoxication include**

   A respiratory alkalosis
   B metabolic acidosis
   C hyperkalaemia
   D hyponatraemia
   E sodium retention

.70. **You are called to see a woman of 35 who has been stung by a bee and who has collapsed. The following considerations should guide your management:**

   A if she has never had an adverse reaction to a sting before, there is no danger to life
   B prompt administration of steroids may be life-saving
   C adrenaline should be given parenterally
   D antihistamines have no place in the treatment
   E following recovery, desensitisation with bee venom is advisable

71. **In acute poisoning with digoxin**

   A potassium supplements should not be given until the serum potassium is known
   B ventricular ectopic beats, without other abnormality, should not be treated unless cardiac output is impaired
   C forced diuresis is essential
   D gastric lavage is dangerous
   E atropine may reduce or abolish ventricular ectopic beats

72. **Manifestations of poisoning by organophosphate insecticides include**

   A dilatation of the pupils
   B blurred vision
   C muscular rigidity
   D hypersalivation
   E glycosuria

73. In the case of a subject with a recessive disorder

A the abnormal gene is present in one or other parent but not both
B the probability of the parents producing a further affected child is 1 in 4
C three out of every 4 healthy children will be heterozygous for the abnormal gene
D the likelihood of finding consanguinity in the parents is greatest when the condition is very rare
E the carrier state cannot be detected by clinical examination

74. Antinuclear antibodies may be found in patients suffering from

A rheumatoid arthritis
B primary Sjögren's disease
C fibrosing alveolitis
D chronic active hepatitis
E drug-induced SLE

75. The following are correct statements about genetic abnormalities:

A Down's syndrome is an example of triploidy
B most individuals with an extra sex chromosome are clinically normal
C meiotic non-disjunction causes mosaicism
D single gene defects carried on the X chromosome are usually recessive
E if the same congenital abnormality is found in a brother and sister, the inheritance is probably autosomal recessive

76. The following are transmitted by autosomal dominant inheritance:

A tuberous sclerosis
B cystic fibrosis
C sickle-cell anaemia
D polyposis coli
E dystrophia myotonica

_ **77.** **Vasculitis affects mainly arterioles and venules in**

    A Wegener's granulomatosis
    B mid-line granuloma
    C polymyalgia rheumatica
    D polyarteritis nodosa
    E Behçet's disease

78. **The following are correct statements about scleroderma:**

    A it is more common in women than in men
    B about 75% of all cases show some neurological involvement if this is sought diligently
    C renal involvement implies a poor prognosis
    D the ESR is invariably raised
    E antinuclear antibodies occur in some 60% of cases

79. **In polymyalgia rheumatica**

    A men are more often affected than women
    B the presence of fever rules out the diagnosis
    C the serum alkaline phosphatase is commonly raised
    D treatment with non-steroidal anti-inflammatory drugs often gives satisfactory control
    E treatment should be continued for a minimum of 6 months

80. **In the management of systemic lupus erythematosus**

    A pregnancy must be avoided at all costs
    B chloroquine is valuable in mild cases
    C combined oral contraceptives often suppress disease activity
    D renal biopsy provides important prognostic information in patients with renal involvement
    E the best index of disease activity is the level of circulating immune complexes

81. In toxic multinodular goitre

  A the usual cause is oversecretion of TSH
  B thyroid hormone levels are usually only slightly raised
  C cardiac complications are common
  D the gland is relatively resistant to radio-therapy
  E the treatment of choice is with antithyroid drugs

82. In atrial fibrillation due to hyperthyroidism

  A the serum T4 level is always raised above the upper limit of normal
  B digoxin has little effect on the ventricular rate
  C propranolol is ineffective
  D the administration of anticoagulants is unnecessary
  E control of the hyperthyroidism is followed by reversion to regular rhythm in more than 50% of patients

83. Medication suitable for the treatment of hyperthyroid crisis includes

  A intravenous propranolol
  B oral Lugol's iodine
  C intravenous carbimazole
  D dexamethasone
  E radioactive iodine

84. Recognised manifestations of hypothyroidism include

  A pericardial effusion
  B erythema ab igne
  C amenorrhoea
  D cerebellar ataxia
  E normochromic, normocytic anaemia

85. In Hashimoto's thyroiditis

  A presentation is commonest in the sixth decade
  B the goitre is usually nodular
  C thyroid antibodies are present in high titres
  D treatment with thyroxine usually causes the goitre to shrink
  E the patient is nearly always hypothyroid when first seen

86.   In myxoedema coma

A   convulsions are not uncommon
B   the protein content of the CSF is raised
C   the mortality rate is about 50%
D   the first step in treatment should be an intravenous injection of T3
E   in the absence of clinical evidence of primary hypothyroidism, hydrocortisone should be given intravenously

87.   In patients with a prolactinoma

A   the usual presentation is with infertility
B   if male, the cause is usually a macro-adenoma
C   the onset is earlier in males than in females
D   serum prolactin levels over 1000 mIU/l are diagnostic
E   treatment with bromocriptine will lower prolactin levels but will not affect tumour size

88.   In the interpretation of thyroid function tests the following points are important and true:

A   a rise of more than 1 mU/l in TSH level 20 minutes after the injection of TRH excludes hyperthyroidism
B   seriously ill patients may have plasma T4 levels in the hypothyroid range and yet in fact be euthyroid
C   administration of propranolol may cause abnormally high plasma T3 levels
D   screening of neonates for hypothyroidism is ineffective
E   screening of elderly patients by basal TSH and by total and free T4 desirable

89.   In primary aldosteronism

A   a plasma potassium of 3.6 mmol/l makes the diagnosis exceedingly unlikely
B   severe symptoms are uncommon
C   urinary potassium excretion is inappropriately low
D   basal plasma aldosterone and renin activity is a valuable diagnostic aid
E   due to adrenal hyperplasia the treatment of choice is surgery

90. **Oestrogen therapy for menopausal symptoms is contraindicated in the presence of**

    A severe liver disease
    B heavy smoking
    C uterine fibroids
    D diabetes
    E hypertension

91. **Biochemical changes usually found in patients with polycystic ovary syndrome include**

    A decreased LH:FSH ratio in the early follicular phase
    B increased testosterone levels
    C increased androstenedione levels
    D increased oestrone levels
    E decreased oestradiol levels

92. **In the investigation of a case of hypercalcaemia**

    A failure of a corticosteroid to suppress the hypercalcaemia rules out a malignant cause
    B a raised serum chloride level is suggestive of primary hyperparathyroidism
    C administration of thiazides or lithium is not an adequate explanation of severe hypercalcaemia
    D a low serum inorganic phosphorus level strongly suggests primary hyperparathyroidism
    E a normal plasma PTH level rules out primary hyperparathyroidism

93. **The following drugs can cause gynaecomastia:**

    A cyproterone acetate
    B tamoxifen
    C cyclophosphamide
    D imipramine
    E danazol

94. **A woman of 23 complains of cessation of menstruation for the past 4 months. The serum prolactin level is 1000 mU/l. Possible causes include**

A   pregnancy
B   anorexia nervosa
C   autoimmune ovarian failure
D   prolactin-secreting pituitary adenoma
E   phenothiazine medication

95. **In the investigation and management of infertility**

A   the diagnosis of obstructive azoospermia can only be made on the basis of testicular biopsy
B   even if the woman is having regular menstrual cycles she may not be ovulating
C   examination of the woman's breasts is essential
D   a history of cystic fibrosis in the man indicates probable absence of the vas deferens
E   no effective therapy for varicocele exists

96. **In the investigation of short stature or delayed puberty**

A   measurement of bone age does not assist diagnosis
B   the growth spurt is to be expected early in female puberty but late in male puberty
C   if the child appears normal and is growing at a normal rate no investigations are needed
D   a child suffering from emotional deprivation gives a normal pattern of growth hormone secretion in sleep
E   nearly all children show some sign of pubertal development by their fifteenth birthday

97. **In the diagnosis and management of neuropathic arthropathy in the foot of a diabetic patient**

A   disorganisation of the joint may develop within a few months only
B   warmth over the joint indicates infection and virtually rules out a neuropathic cause
C   early X-rays are likely to be normal
D   the best way of confirming the diagnosis is by bone scan
E   management should include bed rest if possible

98. **Fetal macrosomia**

A   is defined as a birth weight above the 90th centile
B   does not occur in pregnant diabetics if the diabetes is well controlled
C   is best detected during pregnancy by ultrasonic measurement of fetal abdominal size
D   is best managed by conservative obstetrics
E   if encountered unexpectedly at birth is an indication for measurement of the mother's glycosylated haemoglobin

99. **Recognised manifestations of diabetes in children include**

A   growth retardation
B   precocious puberty
C   weight loss
D   increased psychiatric morbidity
E   microvascular disease

100. **In the management of diabetic ketoacidosis**

A   insulin is best given by continuous intravenous infusion
B   any evidence of acidaemia is an indication for bicarbonate administration
C   anticoagulants are absolutely contraindicated
D   a plasma sodium of 150 mmol/l or over is an indication for the infusion of hypotonic saline
E   potassium should not be given until the plasma level has fallen to 4 mmol/l

101. **In non-insulin dependent diabetes**

A   the disease is commoner among males than among females in Europe
B   nearly all identical twins affected have a similarly affected co-twin
C   the islet cells are normal
D   the insulin secreted is of normal biological activity
E   plasma insulin levels are always subnormal

102. **The following are correct statements regarding diabetic nephropathy:**

A   by the time renal function has begun to deteriorate, retinopathy is always present
B   ultrasound examination usually shows diminished renal size
C   the glomerular filtration rate usually declines linearly with time
D   coronary artery disease is rarely a significant problem
E   for end-stage renal failure the preferred treatment is renal transplantation from a live related donor

103. **Recognised causes of fasting hypoglycaemia include**

A   alcoholism
B   retroperitoneal sarcoma
C   pyloroplasty
D   Addison's disease
E   insulinoma

104. **Hypoglycaemia due to sulphonylurea administration**

A   is virtually confined to patients taking chlorpropamide
B   requires hospital admission in all cases
C   has a lower mortality than insulin-induced hypoglycaemia
D   may relapse following an initial response to glucose
E   is best treated by glucagon injection

105. **In the management and prophylaxis of acute porphyrias, the following are indicated:**

A   a reducing diet if the patient is obese
B   morphine if the pain is very severe
C   venesection
D   intravenous haematin
E   β-blocking drugs if hypertension develops

106. **The following examples of hyperlipidaemia characteristically cause the variety of xanthoma mentioned:**

A   familial hypercholesterolaemia: xanthoma tendinosum
B   remnant hyperlipoproteinaemia: palmar xanthomata
C   familial combined hyperlipidaemia: none
D   familial hypertriglyceridaemia: none
E   common hypercholesterolaemia: palmar xanthomata

107. **Characteristic findings on presentation of Fanconi's syndrome include**

A   vomiting
B   alkalosis
C   dehydration
D   fever
E   glycosuria

108. **Hunter's disease can be distinguished from Hurler's disease because in the former**

A   no 'gargoyle-like' facies is found
B   corneal clouding is very uncommon
C   death always occurs before 10 years of age
D   intelligence may be nearly normal
E   transmission is by sex-linked recessive inheritance

109. **In aluminium-related osteodystrophy of renal failure**

A   the serum calcium is usually normal or raised
B   the serum alkaline phosphatase is grossly elevated
C   the serum PTH is usually normal
D   the first item in treatment should be administration of vitamin D
E   aluminium can be removed from the body by administration of desferrioxamine

110. **In Paget's disease of bone**

    A   hypercalcaemia is unusual
    B   urinary excretion of hydroxyproline is increased
    C   serum calcitonin is usually depressed
    D   therapy with calcitonin usually produces symptomatic improvement
    E   therapy with disodium etidronate requires intravenous administration

111. **In osteogenesis imperfecta (Type I)**

    A   transmission is by dominant inheritance
    B   blue sclerae are seen in infancy only
    C   deafness is mainly conductive in origin
    D   the teeth are not affected
    E   aortic incompetence may develop

112. **Metabolic changes resulting from undernutrition include**

    A   impaired utilisation of amino acids released by protein breakdown
    B   decreased total body potassium
    C   decreased total body sodium
    D   decreased total body zinc
    E   impaired resistance to heat stress

113. **Metabolic changes following the ingestion of alcohol include**

    A   increased hepatic production of uric acid
    B   increased hepatic production of lipoproteins
    C   inhibition of the tricarboxylic acid cycle
    D   decreased lactate: pyruvate ratio
    E   decreased hepatic oxidation of fatty acids

114. **Expected clinical chemistry findings in early alcoholic liver disease include**

    A   raised aspartate aminotransferase (AST)
    B   raised alanine aminotransferase (ALT)
    C   raised bilirubin
    D   raised IgA
    E   decreased total protein

115. Wernicke's encephalopathy

    A   occurs only in alcoholics
    B   should not be diagnosed in the absence of ophthalmoplegia
    C   is usually accompanied by peripheral neuropathy
    D   should be treated with large doses of thiamine
    E   may be precipitated by the administration of large amounts of glucose

116. Progressive visual failure due to alcohol abuse

    A   is commoner in heavy smokers
    B   causes loss of colour vision
    C   is not accompanied by any characteristic appearance on retinoscopy
    D   may be arrested by the administration of hydroxocobalamin
    E   is irreversible

117. Recognised findings in alcoholic pseudo-Cushing's syndrome include

    A   proximal muscle wasting
    B   impaired glucose tolerance
    C   raised plasma cortisol
    D   normal suppression of plasma cortisol with dexamethasone
    E   rapid improvement of biochemical abnormalities on withdrawal of alcohol

118. The following are true of blood disorders in alcoholic patients:

    A   the bone marrow in alcoholics with macrocytosis is usually megaloblastic
    B   folate deficiency plays a part in causing a megaloblastic marrow
    C   folate deficiency may be associated with a sideroblastic anaemia
    D   most alcoholics are depleted of iron and should be given routine iron supplements
    E   disseminated intravascular coagulation is a recognised complication of alcoholic liver disease

119. **In acute alcoholic myopathy**

    A pain is unusual
    B the electrocardiogram is likely to show prominent U-waves
    C death may result if the patient continues drinking
    D the serum creatine phosphokinase is raised
    E the affected muscles are swollen

120. **Recognised findings in babies affected by the fetal alcohol syndrome include**

    A microcephaly
    B high birth weight
    C abnormal palmar creases
    D cardiac septal defects
    E deformities of the fingers

121. **The following signs are reliable indications that the cardiac abnormality mentioned is present:**

    A slow rising pulse: aortic stenosis
    B jerky pulse: hypertrophic cardiomyopathy
    C pulsation of the liver: tricuspid regurgitation
    D loud first heart sound: mitral stenosis
    E splitting of the second heart sound: atrial septal defect

122. **In the interpretation of cardiac murmurs the following statements are correct:**

    A a short mid-systolic murmur in the third and second left interspaces is usually innocent
    B the best indication of the severity of mitral stenosis is the loudness of the murmur
    C an immediate diastolic murmur is always due to aortic or pulmonary regurgitation
    D a continuous murmur nearly always indicates a patent ductus arteriosus
    E the tricuspid flow murmur in atrial septal defect is high-pitched

123. **Radiological enlargement of the heart**

    A is best detected by determining the cardiothoracic ratio
    B in conditions causing pressure overload is usually well marked
    C involving the left atrium can be recognised at an early stage
    D involving the left ventricle causes increased prominence of the aortic knuckle
    E in pericardial effusion causes poor definition of the cardiac outline

124. **Cardiac investigations with radioisotopes in normal subjects should reveal**

    A a resting ejection fraction of at least 50%
    B an increase of at least 5 EF units above resting EF on exercise
    C lung uptake significantly higher than myocardial in thallium scanning
    D absence of myocardial uptake in technetium pyrophosphate scans
    E homogeneous uptake in all segments at rest and exercise in thallium scanning

125. Acute pericarditis

A   is most commonly the result of myocardial infarction
B   causes pain which is worse when sitting up
C   nearly always causes characteristic ECG changes
D   may develop within a few hours of myocardial infarction
E   may sometimes be confirmed by echocardiography

126. The following characteristics of chest pain are more suggestive of 'non-specific' pain than of angina pectoris:

A   stabbing quality of the pain
B   radiation to the jaw
C   relief by glyceryltrinitrate within 2 minutes
D   lack of relation to sexual intercourse
E   facilitation by cold or windy weather

127. Pressure measurements within the heart chambers by means of a catheter allow accurate assessment of the severity of

A   mitral stenosis
B   mitral regurgitation
C   pulmonary stenosis
D   tricuspid stenosis
E   aortic regurgitation

128. Accurate measurement of cardiac output

A   requires the use of a cardiac catheter
B   by the Fick principle requires measurement of the oxygen content only of arterial blood
C   by the dye dilution technique requires injection of a bolus of dye into the right atrium
D   by thermodilution requires measurement of the temperature of the blood in the aorta
E   is valuable in assessing early cardiac failure

129. DC cardioversion is the treatment of choice for

A   ventricular fibrillation
B   ventricular tachycardia with hypotension
C   supraventricular tachycardia due to digitalis toxicity
D   lone atrial fibrillation of recent onset
E   atrial flutter of recent onset

130. Fascicular block (hemiblock)

A   always causes gross prolongation of the QRS complex
B   affecting the anterior fascicle causes marked left axis deviation
C   affecting the posterior fascicle causes no change in electrical axis
D   almost invariably progresses within a few months to complete AV block
E   characteristically causes T-wave inversion in lead V1

131. An exercise electrocardiography test should be halted without qualification if

A   the ECG shows 3 or more consecutive ventricular premature beats
B   the ECG shows ST segment depression of over 2 mm
C   the blood pressure falls
D   the patient becomes pale
E   the patient shows gross uncoordination

132. The following electrocardiographic findings are compatible with normal health:

A   frequent extrasystoles in a pregnant woman
B   axis deviation of -45°
C   ST segment elevation without Q waves
D   T wave inversion in leads V2 and V3
E   prominent U waves in anterior chest leads

133. The following are correct statements in connection with the interpretation of electrocardiograms:

A   left ventricular hypertrophy should not be diagnosed on the basis of R and S voltage changes alone

B   a dominant R wave in V1 is a reliable indication of right ventricular hypertrophy

C   right bundle-branch block with a QRS duration greater than 0.12 seconds indicates organic heart disease

D   atrial fibrillation is a common finding in patients with strokes

E   left axis deviation may be associated with obesity

134. The following findings in 24-hour tape ECG recordings must be regarded as requiring further investigation:

A   first degree heart block

B   Wenkebach A-V block

C   brief episodes of atrial fibrillation

D   asystole lasting more than 2 seconds

E   sustained ventricular tachycardia accompanied by symptoms

135. The following are correct statements concerning palpitations:

A   in most patients palpitations are not associated with primary heart disease

B   paroxysmal tachycardias seldom occur on a daily basis

C   paroxysmal atrial fibrillation is very common in the elderly

D   the usual explanation of 'dropped beats' is ectopic activity

E   ectopic beats are commoner when the heart rate is relatively slow

136. Factors predisposing to the development of palpitations include

A   viral infections

B   pregnancy

C   excessive alcohol intake

D   thyrotoxicosis

E   excessive food intake

137. **Surgical intervention in the first year of life is likely to be necessary for all babies with congenital heart disease and**

    A   a packed cell volume greater than 0.65
    B   a clearly defined heart murmur
    C   cyanotic attacks
    D   evidence of coarctation of the aorta
    E   evidence of total anomalous pulmonary venous drainage

138. **The following are correct statements:**

    A   frusemide inhibits closure of a patent ductus arteriosus
    B   prostaglandin infusion may be beneficial in coarctation of the aorta
    C   the drug of choice in neonatal cardiac failure is digoxin
    D   morphine is absolutely contraindicated in the neonate
    E   propranolol reduces the frequency of neonatal cyanotic attacks

139. **In mitral stenosis**

    A   reduction of the mitral orifice to 2.5 cm^2 usually causes severe symptoms
    B   if the valve is rigid the opening snap is absent
    C   digoxin should not be given unless atrial fibrillation has developed
    D   cardiac catheterisation is unnecessary except in special circumstances
    E   anticoagulant treatment is necessary for virtually all patients

140. **In chronic aortic regurgitation**

    A   if there are no symptoms the prognosis is excellent
    B   a systolic ejection murmur indicates accompanying stenosis
    C   end-systolic volume is increased
    D   chest X-ray always reveals cardiomegaly
    E   if symptoms develop medical treatment should be used to postpone valve replacement

141. **Ejection clicks in congenital heart disease may be heard in patients with**

    A   bicuspid aortic valve
    B   aortic valve stenosis
    C   subvalvar aortic stenosis with a normal aortic valve
    D   severe pulmonary stenosis
    E   pulmonary atresia

142. **Innocent cardiac murmurs in children**

    A   are never diastolic
    B   are never continuous
    C   may vary with respiration
    D   are not affected by change in posture
    E   are heard over a limited area

143. **In planning surgery for a patient with valvular heart disease, the following are correct:**

    A   rheumatic aortic stenosis always requires valve replacement
    B   where facilities are available, open valvotomy for mitral stenosis gives better results than the closed operation
    C   the only satisfactory operation for mitral regurgitation is valve replacement
    D   homograft or xenograft valve replacements deteriorate more slowly in younger patients
    E   thromboembolism is more common after aortic than after mitral valve replacement

144. **The following are correct statements regarding rheumatic fever and rheumatic heart disease:**

    A   about 1 in 3 patients with rheumatic fever develop rheumatic heart disease
    B   mitral regurgitation is incompatible with a normal life span
    C   aortic stenosis develops more slowly than aortic regurgitation
    D   the mitral valve is affected in about 60% of patients with rheumatic heart disease
    E   tricuspid valve disease is always accompanied by a mitral valve lesion

145. Hypertension (as defined by the WHO criteria) is virtually non-existent among

A Bushmen
B Bahamians
C Iranian nomads
D North Eastern Japanese
E Amazon basin Indians

146. In the investigation of hypertension it is important to remember that

A adequate urine microscopy will almost always permit a correct diagnosis of glomerulonephritis
B if urine microscopy indicates glomerulonephritis then renal biopsy should be performed
C at least 50% of patients with malignant hypertension have underlying renal disease
D erythrocyte casts in the urine are a certain indication of renal disease
E most cases of polycystic disease of the kidney are only recognised after intravenous urography

147. In the management of hypertension

A a patient with malignant hypertension should be admitted to hospital
B malignant hypertension is an absolute indication for parenteral therapy
C the drug of choice for urgent reduction of blood pressure is sodium nitroprusside
D if left ventricular failure is present, the best drug is labetalol
E diazoxide should be avoided in patients with ischaemic heart disease

148. There is now clear evidence of the effectiveness of

A aspirin in the prevention of strokes
B dipyramidole in the prevention of strokes
C sulphinpyrazone in the prevention of thrombosis on prosthetic heart valves
D fibrinolytic agents in the management of acute myocardial infarction
E aspirin in the prevention of thromboembolism in atrial fibrillation

149. **In the diagnosis of venous thrombosis in the leg**

A clinical symptoms and signs allow a firm diagnosis in some 85% of cases

B if venography is the only confirmatory test available, it should be performed on all patients with suggestive clinical findings

C impedance plethysmography may give false-negative but not false-positive results

D Doppler ultrasound is the best confirmatory test for calf vein thrombosis

E radioiodine fibrinogen scanning should not be used as the only confirmatory test

150. **In the treatment of pulmonary embolism accompanying deep vein thrombosis**

A the intitial heparin therapy is best given by intermittent intravenous injection

B heparin may be discontinued three days after starting oral warfarin therapy

C long-term (3-6 months) warfarin therapy offers no therapeutic advantage

D warfarin must not be given to pregnant women

E the commonest complication of warfarin therapy is bleeding

151. **In patients with cor pulmonale**

A the commonest cause is obstructive airways disease

B the prognosis is relatively good if the cause is pulmonary sarcoidosis

C long-term oxygen therapy has been shown to be ineffective

D digitalis is of doubtful usefulness

E vasodilators are of little value

152. **A patient is referred with a provisional diagnosis of thromboangiitis obliterans (Buerger's disease). You would feel inclined to reject this diagnosis if you found**

A the patient was a male

B symptoms were confined to the legs

C the patient was not Jewish

D the patient was a non-smoker

E both femoral pulses were impalpable

153. **Relatively higher rates of ischaemic heart disease are seen in**

A   Scotland compared with Japan
B   south east England compared with north England
C   manual workers in developed countries
D   professional classes in developing countries
E   Greece compared with Finland

154. **The following are correct statements about the medical treatment of angina:**

A   the action of sublingual isosorbide dinitrate lasts longer than that of sublingual glyceryl trinitrate
B   bradycardia is a reliable index of adequate dosage of a β-blocker
C   diltiazem produces vasodilatation without tachycardia
D   verapamil slows conduction through the A-V node
E   the drug of choice in Prinzmetal's angina is nifedipine

155. **In angina of increasing severity ('unstable angina')**

A   hospital admission is desirable
B   β-blockers are contraindicated
C   the patient should have a supply of sublingual nitrates
D   intravenous nitrate therapy can only be used if blood nitrate levels can be measured
E   oral aspirin reduces the incidence of subsequent infarction

156. **There is firm evidence that mortality in myocardial infarction can be reduced by the administration of**

A   β-blockers
B   intravenous nitroglycerine
C   nifedipine
D   verapamil
E   intravenous streptokinase

157. **The following are appropriate procedures when managing arrhythmias following cardiac infarction:**

   A   R on T extrasystoles: administration of lignocaine
   B   ventricular extrasystoles in runs of more than 3 beats: intravenous procainamide
   C   atrial fibrillation: cardioversion
   D   high-grade AV block following anterior infarction: insertion of pacemaker
   E   sinus bradycardia at less than 40 beats per minute: intravenous atropine

158. **There is clear evidence that the risk of a recurrence of myocardial infarction can be reduced by**

   A   stopping smoking
   B   lowering serum cholesterol
   C   controlling hypertension
   D   reduction of obesity
   E   use of anticoagulants

159. **When a patient with myocardial infarction is admitted to hospital, the risk of death during that admission is increased by**

   A   increasing age of the patient
   B   history of a previous infarction
   C   inferior rather than anterior infarction on ECG
   D   bradycardia on admission
   E   low blood pressure

160. **Useful prognostic information following cardiac infarction can be obtained from**

   A   a return (or not) to normal of the ECG
   B   exercise testing
   C   measurement of ejection fraction
   D   the repetitive ventricular response
   E   prolonged ECG monitoring

161. **The dose of warfarin may need to be reduced if any of the following drugs are given in addition:**

   A   cimetidine
   B   chloramphenicol
   C   sulphinpyrazone
   D   cholestyramine
   E   rifampicin

162. **Infective endocarditis**

   A   is more likely to occur in severely deformed valves than in those with mild abnormalities
   B   in patients with valvular abnormalities is most commonly associated with a congenital bicuspid aortic valve
   C   is uncommon in atrial septal defect
   D   is decreasing in incidence in developed countries
   E   develops on a background of previously diagnosed heart disease in some 85% of cases

163. **In infective endocarditis**

   A   the organism most commonly responsible in general medical patients is *Streptococcus viridans*
   B   emboli are usually sterile
   C   the C3-complement level is nearly always reduced
   D   nephritis may cause impairment of renal function
   E   treatment should be started as soon as the clinical suspicion arises without waiting for bacteriological confirmation

164. **In fungal infective endocarditis**

   A   the infecting organism is usually *Candida*
   B   the infection is never primary
   C   the vegetations are usually small and wart-like
   D   blood cultures are nearly always positive
   E   chemotherapy will usually effect a complete cure

165. **In the treatment of heart failure with vasodilator drugs**

    A   the ventricular filling pressure decreases
    B   the cardiac output increases
    C   the cardiac oxygen consumption increases
    D   symptomatic relief is proportional to the rise in cardiac output
    E   adverse reactions are particularly common in the presence of hyponatraemia

166. **In aortic dissection**

    A   syncope may occur
    B   the blood pressure is normal or elevated
    C   plasma levels of cardiac enzymes are normal
    D   if the ascending aorta is involved, immediate surgery is essential
    E   if the ascending aorta is not involved, lowering the blood pressure by means of drugs is likely to be successful

167. **In pericardial effusion with tamponade**

    A   diastolic pressures are high in all four cardiac chambers
    B   the arterial pulse pressure is low
    C   relief of symptoms by aspiration occurs only after about 50% of the fluid has been removed
    D   the venous pressure rises on inspiration
    E   there is overloading of the ventricles

168. **In constrictive pericarditis**

    A   there is gross enlargement of the liver
    B   an enlarged spleen would suggest that hepatic cirrhosis was a more likely diagnosis
    C   a systolic murmur is unsually audible at the base of the heart
    D   the ECG shows low voltages
    E   echocardiography shows enlargement of the atria

169. A woman aged 30 is referred with a provisional diagnosis of rheumatoid arthritis. You would be inclined to discard this if you found

A   a history of tingling in the hands at night
B   a painless, red eye
C   a pericardial effusion
D   a palpable spleen
E   generalised lymphadenopathy

170. Recognised laboratory findings in rheumatoid arthritis include

A   presence of antinuclear factor
B   increased DNA binding
C   increased platelet count
D   elevated serum alkaline phosphatase
E   elevated serum C-reactive protein

171. Recognised radiological findings in osteoarthritis include

A   juxta-articular osteoporosis
B   soft tissue swelling
C   bone cysts
D   subchondral bone sclerosis
E   subchondral bone remodelling

172. In suspected septic arthritis

A   the most important procedure is joint aspiration
B   no diagnostic decision should be taken until the results of culture are known
C   a negative culture rules out gonococcal infection
D   surgical drainage is nearly always necessary
E   mobilisation of the joint should begin as soon as symptoms allow

173. Acute iridocyclitis commonly causes

A   lacrimation
B   photophobia
C   blurred vision
D   dilatation of the pupil
E   hypopyon

174. The following are correct statements:

A   the HLA-B27 antigen is found in about 1% of white subjects
B   the HLA-B27 antigen is more common in white subjects than in blacks
C   over 95% of patients with primary ankylosing spondylitis are HLA-B27 positive
D   patients with psoriatic arthropathy give a negative response to tests for rheumatoid factor
E   randomly selected individuals with HLA-B27 have a 2-10% chance of developing spondylitis

175. In juvenile rheumatoid arthritis

A   the incidence is greater in girls than in boys
B   subcutaneous nodules are uncommon
C   the hands and feet are affected first
D   the latex test is usually positive
E   if activity of the disease persists into adult life there is considerable risk of serious disability

176. In systemic juvenile chronic arthritis

A   diagnosis depends mainly on laboratory tests
B   leucopenia is usual
C   onset is usually in infancy
D   joint manifestations are absent at onset
E   there is continuous fever

177. The propionic acid group of NSAIDs includes

    A   ibuprofen
    B   naproxen
    C   tiaprofenic acid
    D   mefenamic acid
    E   diclofenac

178. Improvement in pregnancy is usual in

    A   rheumatoid arthritis
    B   systemic lupus erythematosus
    C   ankylosing spondylitis
    D   systemic sclerosis
    E   dermatomyositis

179. In acute gout

    A   fever is common
    B   the first attack is nearly always monarticular
    C   the plasma urate is always raised
    D   the synovial fluid may be purulent
    E   the drug of choice is indomethacin

180. In the treatment of rheumatoid arthritis with gold, the drug should be discontinued if

    A   there is no response after a total of 500 mg has been given
    B   the WBC count falls below 4000×10^9 /l
    C   the urine shows a trace of protein
    D   a skin rash develops
    E   hepatitis develops

181. In the treatment of rheumatoid arthritis with penicillamine, the drug should be discontinued if

    A   there is no response after the dose has been raised to 1000 mg daily
    B   a pemphigus-like rash develops
    C   the patient loses the sense of taste
    D   the platelet count falls to less than $40,000 \times 10^9$ /l
    E   nausea and vomiting develop

182. **Organisms known to produce enteropathic reactive arthritis include**

A *Brucella melitensis*
B *Salmonella typhimurium*
C *Shigella flexneri*
D *Shigella sonnei*
E *Campylobacter* spp

183. **In enteropathic arthritis complicating inflammatory bowel disease**

A the joint most commoly affected is the knee
B there are marked destructive changes in the affected joints
C the incidence is reduced by control of the gut disease
D local injection of corticosteroids should be avoided
E non-steroidal anti-inflammatory agents are beneficial

184. **Characteristic features of familial Mediterranean fever include**

A autosomal recessive inheritance
B abdominal pain
C a bullous skin eruption
D asymmetric arthritis
E effective prevention of attacks by prophylactic colchicine

185. The risk of gastric cancer is increased in subjects who

A have a first degree relative with gastric cancer
B are of blood group B
C are heavy cigarette smokers
D consume substantial amounts of dairy produce
E consume substantial amounts of fresh vegetables

186. The following are correct statements:

A autoimmune chronic gastritis causes atrophic gastritis but not intestinal metaplasia
B hypersecretory chronic gastritis does not involve an increased risk of gastric cancer
C environmental chronic gastritis carries an increased risk of gastric cancer
D gastric mucosal dysplasia is a pre-cancerous condition
E completely differentiated gastric intestinal metaplasia is a pre-cancerous condition

187. Recognised causes of constipation include

A lead poisoning
B hyperkalaemia
C hypercalcaemia
D Chagas' disease
E porphyria

188. Heartburn

A is always felt behind the lower end of the sternum
B does not radiate to the back
C may be precipitated by alcohol
D is a recognised feature of peptic ulceration
E may follow the reflux of neutral gastric juice

189. A patient is referred with a provisional diagnosis of 'nervous dyspepsia'. You would be suspicious of an organic cause if you found a history of

A morning nausea
B early satiety
C inability to eat for several hours after vomiting
D loss of weight
E painless diarrhoea

190. In gastric ulceration

A gastric acid production is greatly increased
B the patient is more commonly of upper socio-economic class
C perforation is less common than in duodenal ulceration
D a once daily bedtime dose of an H_2-receptor antagonist is satisfactory treatment
E maintenance treatment after healing with an H_2-receptor antagonist will delay recurrence

191. In osmotic diarrhoea

A the total ionic concentration of the stool exceeds the measured osmolality by more than 50 mmol/l
B a 48-hour fast may be expected to reduce the diarrhoea
C a non-absorbed solute should be sought
D laxative abuse can be ruled out
E the cause may be lactase deficiency

192. In gastro-oesophageal reflux

A mucosal pain does not occur in the absence of oesophagitis
B a rolling hiatus hernia is a common cause
C antacid therapy is ineffective once oesophagitis has developed
D standard treatment with cimetidine will nearly always heal oesophagitis
E surgery is only rarely successful in controlling the reflux

193. **In acute upper gastrointestinal haemorrhage**

    A the advent of fibre-optic endoscopy has reduced the overall mortality rate from 10% to less than 5%

    B transfusion is required if the haemoglobin on admission is less than 10 g/dl

    C if oesophageal varices are suspected, urgent endoscopy is required

    D bed rest and sedation have been clearly shown to be beneficial

    E in patients with duodenal ulcer, cimetidine is effective in stopping bleeding

194. **Secretory IgA**

    A contains a dimer of IgA

    B is protected against digestive proteases

    C can neutralise viruses

    D requires the presence of complement for its effect

    E promotes the absorption of antigens

195. **Food intolerance**

    A is caused by non-immunological mechanisms

    B does not produce urticaria or asthma

    C may involve the activation of complement

    D is more common than food allergy in adults

    E is dose-dependent

196. **Immunoproliferative small intestinal disease**

    A is particularly common among Sephardic Jews

    B does not occur in the southern hemisphere

    C is painless

    D may cause complete loss of intestinal villi

    E may respond to radiotherapy

197. In gluten-sensitive enteropathy

    A   constipation rules out the diagnosis
    B   many adults do not have a childhood history
    C   in children, a third biopsy after gluten challenge is essential
    D   the diet must exclude wheat, rye and barley
    E   in severely ill patients, prednisolone should be included in the initial treatment

198. In parenteral nutrition

    A   the preferred route is via a catheter in the superior vena cava
    B   calories in excess of requirements given as carbohydrate are stored as hepatic glycogen
    C   when intravenous fat is given the glucose input should be increased
    D   carbohydrate infusion increases sodium retention
    E   optimum nitrogen balance requires the addition of magnesium to the infusion

199. Recognised symptoms in irritable bowel syndrome include

    A   a sense of incomplete defaecation
    B   passage of mucus per rectum
    C   rectal bleeding
    D   a sense of abdominal distension
    E   loss of weight

200. Recognised findings in patients with VIPomas include

    A   watery diarrhoea
    B   hyperkalaemia
    C   acidosis
    D   occasional normal fasting plasma VIP levels
    E   resistance to chemotherapy

201. In the examination of the rectum and sigmoid colon

A the optimum diameter of the sigmoidoscope is 1 cm

B rectal perforation following biopsy will almost certainly lead to peritonitis

C sigmoidoscopy should not be performed in the presence of a bleeding diathesis

D a barium enema should not be performed within 48 hours of rectal biopsy

E anal Crohn's disease may make digital examination of the rectum completely impossible

202. Recognised causes of occult or minor overt rectal bleeding include

A anal Crohn's disease

B angiodysplasia

C colonic diverticular disease

D pseudo-membranous colitis

E tubo-villous adenoma of the colon

203. Histological features favouring ulcerative colitis rather than Crohn's disease include

A depleted goblet cells

B granulomas

C thickened muscularis mucosae

D heavy submucosal inflammation

E widespread crypt abscesses

204. In ulcerative colitis

A pregnancy will almost certainly precipitate a relapse

B if the disease is limited to the left colon the increased risk of cancer is slight

C the prognosis of individual attacks worsens with increasing age

D sulphasalazine should be given for at least 1 year after the first episode

E broad-spectrum antibiotics are a useful adjunct to sulphasalazine

205. In diverticulitis of the colon

A the best clue to the diagnosis is the radiological appearance
B when diarrhoea is the main symptom, bran may be ineffective
C morphine should be avoided
D peritonitis may develop
E metronidazole is absolutely contraindicated

206. Antibiotic-related colitis

A is rarely due to treatment with lincomycin
B is more likely to develop the longer the antibiotic is given
C is more likely to develop in older patients
D can be confirmed by laboratory examination of a stool sample
E is best treated with oral metronidazole

207. Recognised manifestations of Crohn's disease include

A iritis
B erythema annulare centrifugum
C massive bowel haemorrhage
D nocturnal diarrhoea
E finger clubbing

208. In Crohn's disease in children

A diffuse small bowel involvement is more common than in adults
B a pattern of recurrent attacks is unusual
C stricture formation may cause retardation of growth
D corticosteroid therapy is contraindicated
E surgery should if possible be postponed until the patient is fully grown

209. In the management of chronic pancreatitis it is usually necessary to provide parenteral replacement of

A calciferol
B vitamin K
C vitamin C
D vitamin B_{12}
E vitamin B_6

210. Carcinoma of the pancreas

    A   affects women twice as commonly as men
    B   is more likely to occur in West Indian negroes than in whites
    C   causing pain is usually inoperable
    D   does not respond to chemotherapy
    E   responds to radiotherapy in some 30-40% of patients

211. Recognised causes of acute pancreatitis include

    A   hyperlipaemia
    B   hypocalcaemia
    C   infection with Coxsackie B virus
    D   treatment with azathioprine
    E   infection with *Mycoplasma pneumoniae*

212. The following pathological changes occur in cystic fibrosis:

    A   impaired reabsorption of chloride from sweat
    B   impaired reabsorption of bicarbonate from pancreatic juice
    C   impaired secretion of chloride in the lungs
    D   focal areas of biliary cirrhosis in the liver
    E   dilated crypts in the intestine

213. Recognised complications of cystic fibrosis include

    A   rectal prolapse
    B   metabolic acidosis
    C   gall stones
    D   cirrhosis of the liver
    E   pancreatitis

214. In familial Mediterranean fever

    A   the disease does not occur before puberty
    B   recurrent attacks of arthritis are likely to cause permanent joint damage
    C   the ESR is nearly always raised during an attack
    D   amyloidosis is uncommon in Jewish patients
    E   colchicine reduces the frequency and severity of the attacks

215. Eosinophilic infiltration of the gut

A is usually associated with eosinophilia of the peripheral blood
B is commonest in the sigmoid colon
C usually presents with the formation of sinuses
D should not be treated with corticosteroids
E may respond to sodium cromoglycate

216. The following are correct statements:

A bacterial culture is essential for the confirmation of suspected rectal gonorrhoea
B lymphogranuloma venereum is best treated with metronidazole
C homosexual men run a particular risk of infection with non-A non-B hepatitis
D enteric symptoms in a homosexual male with normal sigmoidoscopic findings suggest *Giardia lamblia* infection
E the usual cause of death in Kaposi's sarcoma is bone-marrow failure

217. **Mucoceles**

    A   are the result of viral infection
    B   are fluctuant
    C   characteristically develop slowly over many years
    D   are best treated by incision and drainage
    E   may respond to cryosurgery

218. **Sjögren's syndrome**

    A   is more common in women than in men
    B   is usually progressive
    C   is not associated with malignancy
    D   is commonly associated with salivary gland enlargement
    E   is often associated with accelerated dental caries

219. **Results of liver function tests on a patient show: (1) gross elevation of alanine aminotransferase, (2) slight elevation of alkaline phosphatase, (3) normal serum bilirubin. These findings are suggestive of**

    A   chronic persistent hepatitis
    B   chronic active hepatitis
    C   acute hepatitis
    D   hepatic cirrhosis
    E   hepatic malignancy

220. **Non-A, non-B hepatitis**

    A   is now known to be due to a virus of the echovirus group
    B   is associated with a carrier state
    C   has an incubation period of 60-180 days
    D   commonly does not cause jaundice
    E   carries no risk of subsequent cirrhosis

221. **In treatment of acute hepatitis due to hepatitis A virus**

A the patient should be nursed in isolation for 10 days after the appearance of jaundice
B strict bed-rest during this period is advisable
C careful dietary control is necessary
D drugs should be avoided unless absolutely necessary
E the period of convalescence should be approximately twice the symptomatic period

222. **In fulminant hepatic failure**

A encephalopathy always occurs
B hepatitis A is never the cause
C due to administration of halothane, mortality of at least 80% may be expected
D falling levels of serum aminotransferases portend clinical improvement
E acidosis is usual in the early stages

223. **The following findings in and around the mouth may be indicative of the conditions named:**

A retarded dental eruption: Down's syndrome
B epulis: pregnancy
C bleeding gums: use of oral contraceptives
D oral purpura: amyloidosis
E swelling of lips: Crohn's disease

224. **Recurrent aphthous ulceration of the mouth**

A has been shown to have an autoimmune basis in some patients
B has no hereditary basis
C may remit during pregnancy
D is significantly associated with food intolerance
E is commonly precipitated or aggravated by smoking

225. **In chronic persistent hepatitis**

    A there are no symptoms or physical signs
    B serum AST and ALT levels are normal
    C the serum bilirubin level is normal
    D the serum immunoglobulin level is nearly always raised
    E progression to cirrhosis does not occur

226. **Autoimmune chronic active hepatitis**

    A is genetically determined
    B is more common in females
    C is only rarely accompanied by other autoimmune disorders
    D usually causes a rise in serum IgG levels
    E should be treated with prednisolone

227. **In the investigation of liver disease**

    A the first investigation in suspected acute cholecystitis should be scintigraphy
    B a normal common bile duct cannot be seen on CT scanning
    C technetium-labelled colloid is selectively taken up by liver tumours
    D very small amounts of ascites can be detected by ultrasound
    E in Budd-Chiari syndrome scintigraphy gives a characteristic appearance

228. **In primary biliary cirrhosis**

    A liver biopsy is usually diagnostic
    B asymptomatic patients may have a normal or near normal life expectancy
    C immunosuppressive agents constitute the treatment of choice
    D corticosteroids should not be given on a long-term basis
    E the main bone disorder is osteomalacia

229. **In the control of bleeding from oesophageal varices**

    A   patients with intrahepatic portal hypertension have a poorer prognosis than those with presinusoidal variety

    B   before vasopressin is given, an ECG must be taken

    C   a Sengstaken-Blakemore balloon may be left inflated for up to 48 hours

    D   a single endoscopic injection of sclerosant will stop the bleeding in 70% of patients

    E   β-blocking drugs should not be given

230. **The following are correct statements:**

    A   patients with hepatocellular carcinoma nearly always have jaundice on presentation

    B   cholangiocarcinomas do not produce α-fetoprotein

    C   hepatocellular carcinomas are resistant to radiotherapy

    D   the commonest hepatic tumour in children is hepatoblastoma

    E   the commonest benign hepatic tumour is hepatocellular adenoma

231. **In the screening and management of relatives of a patient with haemochromatosis**

    A   liver biopsy should be performed in siblings with an HLA status identical to that of the proband

    B   the definitive test is the identification of a deficiency of ferritin transferase

    C   alcoholic liver disease can usually be distinguished on the basis of hepatic iron concentration

    D   venesection should be repeated weekly until the haemoglobin concentration falls below 11 g/dl

    E   therapy is not usually needed after the age of 55 to 60

232. **Gallstones**

    A   have a prevalence of over 50% in subjects over 65 years of age

    B   are more likely in subjects taking a diet with a high fibre content

    C   are usually symptomless

    D   are nearly always radio-opaque

    E   respond poorly to medical therapy

AIDS AND SEXUALLY TRANSMITTED DISEASES

233. **In acute LAV/HTLV-III disease**

A the onset is insidious
B the symptoms precede sero-conversion
C there is generalised lymphadenopathy
D lymphocytosis is usual
E the number of suppressor T cells is increased immediately afterwards

234. **In Kaposi's sarcoma occurring in AIDS patients**

A there is a preponderance in homosexual males
B there is early involvement of lymph nodes and viscera
C the gastrointestinal tract is spared
D a diffuse pneumonitis may occur
E there is evidence of a genetic predisposition

235. **The following are common causes of opportunistic infection in patients with AIDS in the UK:**

A cytomegalovirus
B *Pneumocystis carinii*
C *Cryptococcus neoformans*
D *Histoplasma capsulatum*
E *Toxoplasma gondii*

236. **The following are correct statements:**

A both AIDS and persistent generalised lymphadenopathy are uniformly fatal
B a patient who is sero-negative six months after exposure may still be a carrier of the AIDS virus
C the absence of HTLV-III antibodies rules out the diagnosis of persistent generalised lymphadenopathy
D the male:female ratio of AIDS cases in Africa approaches unity
E the prognosis for babies born to AIDS-infected mothers is relatively good

237. **The following are correct statements:**

A nearly all patients with AIDS are anergic
B nearly all patients with AIDS have reduced serum levels of gammaglobulin
C the antigen of HLTV-III/LAV is more difficult to detect than that of hepatitis B virus
D the presence of antibody to HLTV-III/LAV implies continued presence of the virus rather than immunity
E HLTV-III/LAV is more labile to disinfectants than hepatitis B virus

238. **Genital herpes**

A is usually caused by herpes simplex virus type 2
B usually has an incubation period of 4-5 days
C characteristically causes a mild first attack, followed by recurrences of increasing severity
D can most accurately be confirmed by cell culture
E is resistant to all anti-viral agents

239. **Gonorrhoea can usually be reliably diagnosed by examination of a Gram-stained smear from**

A the urethral discharge in a male
B the vaginal discharge in a female
C the pharynx
D the rectum
E the haemorrhagic skin pustules in gonococcal bacteraemia

240. **The rash of secondary syphilis**

A usually starts on the face
B spares the palms and the soles
C is more profuse on flexor than extensor surfaces
D is not usually irritant
E is symmetrically distributed

RENAL DISORDERS

241. **Relatively raised levels of serum creatinine are likely to be reported if the patient**

    A is a muscular male
    B is taking aspirin
    C is elderly
    D has been fasting for several days
    E has a grossly increased plasma glucose level

242. **The following biochemical results may be accepted as normal:**

    A plasma chloride 100 mmol/l
    B plasma osmolality 320 mOsmol/kg
    C serum ionized calcium 2.5 mmol/l
    D total serum cholesterol 5 mmol/l
    E serum inorganic phosphate 3.2 mmol/l

243. **Hypertension in pregnancy**

    A is due to underlying renal disease in 50% of women affected
    B due to pre-eclampsia usually recurs in subsequent pregnancies
    C due to lupus nephritis carries a bad prognosis for both mother and baby regardless of treatment
    D due to glomerulonephritis may precipitate a sharp deterioration in renal function
    E due to polycystic disease carries no added risk to mother and baby

244. **The following are correct statements:**

    A a history of asthma implies a greatly increased risk of an adverse reaction to intravenous urography (IUV)
    B low-osmolar, non-ionic contrast agents for IVU give results inferior to those obtained with conventional media
    C radiologically non-opaque calculi cannot be detected by CT scanning
    D a single episode of urinary tract infection in an adult male gives sufficient grounds for requesting an IVU
    E ultrasound is a sensitive procedure for the detection of obstruction of the urinary tract

245. **The following are correct statements:**

A   polyuria due to chronic renal failure seldom exceeds 3 litres/24 hours

B   cloudy urine without symptoms is rarely due to pyuria

C   the smell of the urine is normally of no importance

D   low back pain is an important early symptom in renal disease

E   orthostatic proteinuria may be a manifestation of intrinsic renal disease

246. **Nocturnal enuresis is more likely to occur if the child**

A   is a boy

B   is the youngest in a large family

C   is of social class III or IV

D   has experienced severe stress in early life

E   has a first degree relative who had enuresis

247. **In the use of buzzer alarms in treating nocturnal enuresis**

A   benefit is unlikely until the child is at least 8 years old

B   most children take about 2 months to become dry

C   relapse is uncommon after 42 consecutive dry nights

D   the alarm should be placed as near as possible to the sleeping child

E   the usual cause for a wet bed and a silent alarm is an electrical failure in the alarm system

248. **Recognised causes of urinary incontinence include**

A   previous radiotherapy

B   multiple sclerosis

C   Parkinson's disease

D   diabetic neuropathy

E   faecal impaction

249. **In the assessment of proteinuria discovered unexpectedly at routine examination**

    A   a urinary protein output of over 80 mg/24 hrs is definite evidence of renal disease
    B   a urinary protein output of more than 1g/24 hrs normally requires renal biopsy
    C   proteinuria may persist for years without progressive renal impairment
    D   orthostatic proteinuria is always benign
    E   persistent heavy proteinuria may indicate progressive disease even if the blood pressure and biochemical findings are normal

250. **Deposition of IgG on the glomerular basement membrane is a characteristic pathological finding in**

    A   membranous nephropathy
    B   anti-GBM antibody mediated nephropathy
    C   Berger's disease
    D   Henoch-Schönlein nephritis
    E   diffuse endothelial proliferative glomerulonephritis

251. **The mortality in patients with acute renal failure is particularly high in the presence of**

    A   severe burns
    B   hepatorenal syndrome
    C   non-oliguric acute renal failure
    D   pancreatitis
    E   intra-abdominal sepsis

252. **In renal osteodystrophy**

    A   the onset is earlier in interstitial than in glomerular disease
    B   bone histology reveals both osteomalacia and osteitis fibrosa
    C   the earliest indication is the presence of subperiosteal erosions on X-ray of the phalanges
    D   magnesium hydroxide should not be given
    E   serum calcium levels should be corrected by giving vitamin D_3

253. **In patients with terminal renal failure treated with haemodialysis**

A the rate of blood removal required for successful dialysis is 200 ml/minute

B once a stable dialysis routine is established, dietary restrictions are unnecessary

C dialysis to the appropriate dry weight will usually allow antihypertensive drugs to be stopped

D iron deficiency is almost invariable

E blood transfusion should be avoided for as long as possible

254. **Continuous ambulatory peritoneal dialysis offers the following advantages over haemodialysis:**

A better removal of middle molecular weight solutes

B less rigorous fluid restriction and dietary constraint

C improved growth rates in children

D improved control of hyperlipidaemia

E improved maintenance of haemoglobin level

255. **Antenatal diagnosis in early pregnancy of the following hereditary disorders is possible:**

A Alport's syndrome

B congenital nephrotic syndrome

C infantile polycystic disease of the kidney

D adult polycystic disease of the kidney

E cystine storage disease

256. **In adult polycystic disease of the kidneys**

A inheritance is autosomal dominant

B if there is no evidence by modern imaging techniques of the disease at age 20, the risk that it will develop is less than 1%

C if the liver contains cysts, fatal hepatic failure is the usual outcome

D polycythaemia is a recognised complication

E surgical excision of the cysts is now a worthwhile undertaking

257. **In the investigation of suspected urinary obstruction**

A the initial imaging technique should be ultrasound
B normal ultrasound results rule out acute obstruction
C intravenous urography is of no value in the presence of complete obstruction
D retrograde pyelography requires general anaesthesia
E antegrade pyelography is carried out under local anaesthesia

258. **Post-obstructive diuresis**

A cannot be prevented by giving antidiuretic hormone
B should initially be treated by intravenous replacement with normal saline
C will always subside within seven days
D may cause hypokalaemia
E is particularly common when the obstruction has been partial and bilateral

259. **Recognised effects of nephrotoxicity due to antibiotics include**

A renal papillary necrosis
B acute tubular necrosis
C nephrotic syndrome
D Fanconi's syndrome
E acute nephritic syndrome

260. **The following are correct statements relating to analgesic nephropathy:**

A aspirin is less nephrotoxic than phenacetin or paracetamol
B aspirin and paracetamol are concentrated in the renal medulla
C the primary lesion in analgesic nephropathy is renal papillary necrosis
D the syndrome occurs predominantly in females
E if the patient stops abusing analgesics, improvement in renal function may be expected in 70-80% of cases

261. **Extracorporeal shock wave lithotripsy**

- A may require to be given for up to 60 minutes
- B may cause haematuria
- C does not damage the renal parenchyma
- D depends on relatively simple and cheap apparatus
- E needs no subsequent removal of fragments if the procedure is properly carried out

262. **In urinary tract infection in children**

- A the outcome is usually benign
- B the incidence in boys and girls is equal in the first year of life
- C vesicoureteric reflux (VUR) is present in 30% of cases when first seen
- D patients with VUR when first seen nearly always have established renal scarring
- E no structural abnormality can be demonstrated in half the cases

263. **In the diagnosis and treatment of urinary tract infection in children**

- A nitrite testing is unreliable and should be avoided
- B treatment should be started at once without waiting for information about the drug sensitivity of the organism
- C the drug of choice for initial treatment is co-trimoxazole
- D persistent infection in spite of appropriate drug therapy suggests obstruction
- E an ultrasound scan should be performed in all infants with proven UTI

264. **In reflux nephropathy in adults**

- A vesicoureteric reflux (VUR) can nearly always be demonstrated with a micturating cystogram
- B formation of new focal renal scars is very uncommon
- C most patients progress in a few years to end-stage renal failure
- D pregnancy has a beneficial effect
- E surgical correction of VUR is usually advisable

265. Recognised causes of finger clubbing include

A fibrosing alveolitis
B chronic persistent hepatitis
C atrial myxoma
D Crohn's disease
E pulmonary sarcoidosis

266. Adult respiratory distress syndrome

A carries an overall mortality of about 50%
B characteristically causes no abnormality until several hours after the insult
C even when fully developed, is not accompanied by abnormal physical signs in the chest
D always causes a fall in arterial oxygen tension
E can be prevented or ameliorated by prophylactic corticosteroids

267. An incidence of pneumothorax of 10% or over must be expected following

A aspiration needle biopsy
B drill biopsy
C tru-cut biopsy
D transbronchial biopsy
E open lung biopsy

268. The following results of respiratory function testing would be compatible with a diagnosis of asthma:

A PEFR: reduced
B FEV_1 : reduced
C TLC: reduced
D RV: reduced
E T_L CO: increased

269. **Broncho-alveolar lavage in the following conditions yields neutrophils as the usual non-macrophage inflammatory cells present:**

A   sarcoidosis
B   extrinsic allergic alveolitis
C   connective tissue disorder
D   asbestosis
E   tuberculosis

270. **Broncho-alveolar lavage usually yields pathognomonic material confirmatory of the diagnosis in cases of**

A   sarcoidosis
B   histiocytosis X
C   pulmonary haemosiderosis
D   alveolar proteinosis
E   cryptogenic fibrosing alveolitis

271. **The following drugs carry a particular risk of causing pulmonary damage:**

A   cyclophosphamide
B   azathioprine
C   bleomycin
D   busulphan
E   6-mercaptopurine

272. **Pleural disease is a recognised complication of treatment with**

A   procainamide
B   hydralazine
C   practolol
D   methysergide
E   bromocriptine

273. **The following abnormalities are characteristic of chronic bronchitis:**

    A   enlargement of tracheobronchial mucus glands
    B   enlargement of pulmonary acini
    C   atrophy of bronchial cartilage
    D   loss of pulmonary recoil
    E   excessive numbers of macrophages in respiratory bronchioles

274. **Inheritance of α_1 -antitrypsin activity leads to the following consequences:**

    A   patients homozygous for 'M' protease inhibitor genes (PiM) have normal levels of serum α_1 -antitrypsin
    B   the 'Z' gene is recessive
    C   patients homozygous for the 'Z' gene (PiZ) make up some 50% of those with persistent airflow limitation
    D   patients with the PiZ phenotype are susceptible to a distinctive type of liver disease
    E   heterozygous subjects with the PiMZ phenotype show a clearly increased susceptibility to emphysema

275. **Hepatic metabolism of theophylline is reduced by**

    A   cor pulmonale
    B   tobacco
    C β-blocking drugs
    D   increasing age
    E   ethanol

276. **Cor pulmonale is a recognised complication of**

    A   cystic fibrosis
    B   kyphoscoliosis
    C   filariasis
    D   gross obesity
    E   exposure to high altitude

277. **In long-term domiciliary oxygen therapy for obstructive airways disease with oedema**

A   the oxygen must be given for at least 15 hours per day if survival is to improve

B   no further improvement in survival is gained by prolonging therapy for more than 6 months

C   if an oxygen concentrator is used, the emergent gas contains at least 90% of oxygen

D   the best mode of delivery with an oxygen concentrator is via nasal cannulae

E   no other group of patients has been shown clearly to benefit

278. **Respiration during REM sleep characteristically produces**

A   irregular breathing

B   occasional apnoea or hypopnoea

C   increased sensitivity to hypoxia

D   increased response to bronchopulmonary irritation

E   in patients with cyanotic cor pulmonale ('blue bloaters'), severe oxygen desaturation

279. **A lymphocytic pleural effusion is likely to be due to**

A   pulmonary infarction

B   secondary malignancy of the pleura

C   lymphoma

D   tuberculosis

E   mesothelioma

280. **The following principles should govern the management of spontaneous pneumothorax:**

A   all cases require in-patient care until the pneumothorax is clearly resolving

B   if respiration is embarrassed, treatment can be by aspiration or by intercostal drainage

C   a tension pneumothorax should be released immediately by insertion of an intercostal cannula

D   if more than 2 litres of air is removed a further chest X-ray should be performed

E   a complete pneumothorax must be treated by intercostal drainage

281. **In assessing the prognosis and planning the treatment of a patient with lung cancer, the following are correct:**

    A   the treatment most likely to be curative for non-small cell cancer is surgery

    B   the most radio-sensitive tumour type is small-cell cancer

    C   chemotherapy has no place in the treatment of small-cell cancer

    D   prophylactic cerebral irradiation has been clearly shown to prolong survival in small-cell cancer

    E   chemotherapy after surgery for non-small cell cancer does not prolong survival

282. **In lung cancer**

    A   of the small-cell type, finger clubbing is common

    B   the syndrome of inappropriate secretion of ADH occurs virtually exclusively in the small-cell type

    C   sputum examination is of little value in determining cell-type

    D   bronchial brushing specimens are as accurate as biopsy specimens

    E   hypercalcaemia is most common in squamous-cell tumours

283. **Acute laryngotracheitis**

    A   may be caused by influenza A virus

    B   causes louder stridor than does epiglottitis

    C   causing cyanosis requires hospital admission

    D   responds within a few hours to the administration of corticosteroids

    E   should be treated routinely with broad-spectrum antibiotics

284. **Acute epiglottitis**

    A   is usually due to *Staphylococcus aureus*

    B   is rapid in onset

    C   is characterised by a loud, barking cough

    D   is a medical emergency

    E   should be treated with ampicillin

285. **Secondary chemoprophylaxis (to prevent clinical tuberculosis in infected subjects) is advisable for**

A   infected infants under 5 years old
B   subjects whose tuberculin reaction has recently become positive
C   patients with a history of alcoholism
D   patients receiving long-term corticosteroids
E   Asian immigrants aged 13-14 who are strongly tuberculin-positive

286. **Characteristic features of *Pneumocystis carinii* pneumonia include**

A   absence of fever
B   dry cough
C   conspicuous crackles and wheezes heard at one or other lung base
D   positive blood culture
E   clinical response to co-trimoxazole

287. **Elevation of serum angiotensin-converting enzyme may fail to distinguish pulmonary sarcoidosis from**

A   tuberculosis
B   silicosis
C   cryptogenic fibrosing alveolitis
D   extrinsic allergic alveolitis
E   asbestosis

288. **Characteristic findings in mesothelioma include**

A   chest pain
B   finger clubbing
C   mediastinal shift towards the diseased side
D   poor response to chemotherapy
E   occasional excellent response to radiotherapy

289. **A patient with persistent wheezing is found to have widespread opacities on chest X-ray. The eosinophil count is 3.5 x 10^9 /l. The serum IgE level is grossly raised. You would suspect the presence of**

   A   allergic bronchopulmonary aspergillosis
   B   filariasis
   C   ascariasis
   D   cryptogenic pulmonary eosinophilia
   E   allergic granulomatosis (Churg-Strauss syndrome)

290. **The following laboratory findings are consistent with acute extrinsic allergic alveolitis:**

   A   neutrophilia
   B   raised ESR
   C   eosinophilia
   D   raised serum complement
   E   reduced pulmonary diffusing capacity

291. **Cystic fibrosis**

   A   is the third most important hereditary disease in China
   B   causes recognisable lung disorder at birth
   C   causes disease most commonly in the right upper lobe
   D   leads to increased residual lung volume
   E   requires measles immunisation as early as possible

292. **Asthma may be caused by occupational exposure to**

   A   epoxy resins
   B   fluoride
   C   asbestos
   D   cobalt
   E   colophony

293. **Coal-workers' pneumoconiosis**

   A   carries an increased risk of tuberculosis
   B   is not affected in its course by cigarette smoking
   C   is at present decreasing in the UK
   D   is best controlled by the use of respirators
   E   responds well to low-dosage steroid therapy

294. **In cryptogenic fibrosing alveolitis**

A   the FEV$_1$ is low
B   the FEV$_1$ /FVC ratio is normal or high
C   there is nearly always a polymorph leucocytosis
D   the presence of circulating anti-nuclear factor is very rare
E   lung biopsy is necessary for unequivocal diagnosis

295. **In the management of childhood asthma**

A   skin allergy testing is essential
B   pulmonary function testing is unreliable in children under the age of 8
C   the introduction of non-allergenic pillows and blankets often produces spectacular improvement
D   prevention of bacterial infection with antibiotics is an important means of preventing attacks
E   a child on a maintenance regime of inhaled corticosteroid must have a supply of oral corticosteroid at home

296. **The allergic mechanism involved in the following clinical conditions is of the type specified:**

A   bronchial asthma: Type I
B   Goodpasture's syndrome: Type III
C   farmer's lung: Types III and IV
D   bird-fancier's lung: Type III
E   pulmonary tuberculosis: Type IV

297. Characteristic metabolic changes in patients subjected to trauma include

A   increased hepatic gluconeogenesis
B   inhibition of triglyceride release from adipose tissue
C   increased release of amino acids from muscle
D   increased rate of hepatic synthesis of albumin
E   increased rate of hepatic synthesis of complement

298. In circulatory or septic shock

A   conversion of pyruvate to acetyl co-enzyme A is increased
B   the redox potential declines
C   lactate production increases
D   an intractable lactic acidosis implies a serious prognosis
E   urea excretion increases

299. Septic shock due to Gram-negative bacteria

A   can be clearly distinguished clinically from that caused by other organisms
B   causes decreased pulmonary vascular resistance
C   usually causes peripheral vasodilatation
D   may cause hypothermia
E   should never be treated with corticosteroids

300. Infusions of blood or colloid solutions are usually preferable to crystalloid infusions for resuscitation in

A   acute haemorrhage
B   septicaemia
C   respiratory failure requiring intermittent positive pressure ventilation
D   diabetic ketoacidosis
E   adult respiratory distress syndrome with hypovolaemia

301. **In intermittent positive pressure ventilation**

    A expiration should be assisted by means of negative pressure

    B the preferred inspiratory/expiratory ratio is 2:1

    C the respiratory rate should not exceed 14 per minute

    D if the lungs are healthy, the inspired oxygen concentration should not be increased

    E positive end-expiratory pressure should be reserved for special circumstances

302. **When assisted ventilation is provided in severe acute asthma**

    A the tidal volume should be small

    B the respiratory rate should be slow

    C the inspiratory/expiratory ratio should be 1:1

    D sedation should be avoided

    E additional humidification is needed

303. **Factors tending to reduce intracranial pressure include**

    A hyperbaric oxygen

    B hypoventilation

    C administration of acetazolamide

    D administration of barbiturates

    E lowered serum osmotic pressure

304. **After a head injury**

    A a period of unconsciousness, unaccompanied by any other neurological abnormality, represents functional change without structural damage (concussion)

    B the duration of post-traumatic amnesia exceeds that of unconsciousness

    C absence of any damage to scalp or skull is good evidence that no serious brain damage has occurred

    D with penetration of the skull, consciousness is not necessarily interrupted

    E a fatal outcome is possible even if consciousness is fully regained with complete lucidity

305. Chemotherapy offers a substantial hope of complete cure in

A   carcinoma of the prostate
B   testicular teratoma
C   ovarian carcinoma
D   acute myeloid leukaemia
E   chronic lymphatic leukaemia

306. Chemotherapy is ineffective in

A   hypernephroma
B   carcinoma of the pancreas
C   oat-cell carcinoma of the bronchus
D   malignant melanoma
E   carcinoma of cervix uteri

307. Hypercalcaemia is a recognised consequence of

A   carcinoma of the kidney
B   myelomatosis
C   tumour lysis syndrome
D   treatment with cyclophosphamide
E   ectopic ACTH syndrome

308. Infiltration of the meninges by tumour

A   is more common with leukaemias and lymphomas than with carcinomas
B   may cause mental confusion
C   cannot be demonstrated by CT scanning
D   may not cause the appearance of malignant cells in the CSF even on repeated examination
E   shows no response to any form of therapy

309. CT scanning is of special value in the

A   demonstration of primary gastrointestinal malignancy
B   detection of nodal metastases from pelvic cancers
C   accurate delineation of pulmonary metastases
D   assessment of the results of therapy in Hodgkin's disease
E   assessment of the operability of oat-cell carcinoma

310. **Megavoltage radiotherapy (>1 million eV)**

    A   avoids the skin reactions caused by orthovoltage (250-350kV) therapy

    B   is the treatment of choice for bony metastases

    C   allows accurate calculation of the radiation dose to deep tissues

    D   does not cause hair loss

    E   should not be combined with chemotherapy

311. **Nausea and vomiting are particularly to be expected following the use of**

    A   busulphan

    B   mercaptopurine

    C   cisplatin

    D   bleomycin

    E   hexamethylmelamine

312. **Bone marrow suppression is the dose-limiting side effect of**

    A   cyclophosphamide

    B   busulphan

    C   vinblastine

    D   vincristine

    E   bleomycin

313. **The following are well-substantiated risk factors for cervical carcinoma:**

    A   low age at first intercourse

    B   sexual promiscuity of the patient

    C   sexual promiscuity of the patient's partner

    D   smoking

    E   oral contraception

314. **In the diagnosis and treatment of malignancy in children**

    A   chemotherapy should be given after any necessary surgery and radiotherapy

    B   surgery and chemotherapy can produce complete cure of Wilm's tumour

    C   neuroblastoma can be cured with monoclonal antibody-directed radioisotopes

    D   osteosarcoma is commonest in the long bones

    E   many cases of Hodgkin's disease can be treated satisfactorily with chemotherapy alone

315. **Hodgkin's disease**

    A   involving two or more lymph node regions on the same side of the diaphragm is classified as Stage III

    B   without systemic symptoms is included in the staging subdivision 'A'

    C   involving bone marrow is best diagnosed by needle marrow biopsy

    D   of Stage IV classification should primarily be treated by chemotherapy

    E   in the male treated with MOPP invariably leads to sterility

316. **Characteristic findings in Waldenström's macroglobulinaemia include**

    A   lymphadenopathy

    B   hepatosplenomegaly

    C   bone disease

    D   neurological disorder

    E   hyperviscosity of plasma

317. **Common laboratory findings in chronic granulocytic leukaemia include**

    A   basophilia

    B   raised platelet count

    C   raised neutrophil alkaline phosphatase score

    D   raised serum vitamin B_{12}

    E   lowered serum vitamin B_{12} -binding protein

318. Chronic lymphocytic leukaemia

    A   is the commonest leukaemia in the USA and Europe

    B   is more common in women than in men

    C   is usually caused by malignant transformation of a B lymphocyte

    D   is diagnosed by chance in about 25% of all cases

    E   can now be cured by combined chemotherapy and radiotherapy

319. Hairy cell leukaemia

    A   affects males more than females

    B   is due to proliferation of cells originating from granulocytes

    C   causes splenomegaly

    D   responds well to splenectomy

    E   carries an increased risk of infection by mycobacteria

320. Testicular tumours

    A   are nearly always painful on presentation

    B   should always be staged prior to orchidectomy

    C   should be removed via the scrotum

    D   if seminomatous are very sensitive to radiotherapy

    E   if non-seminomatous should have follow-up chemotherapy

321. The following are correct statements:

A a normal bone marrow can maintain normal haemoglobin levels in the face of a red cell life span of 30 days
B red cell destruction is only rarely both extravascular and intravascular
C damage by complement usually causes intravascular haemolysis
D protein released by haemoglobin destruction is broken down and converted to urea
E urobilinogen excretion is an accurate guide to the rate of haemolysis

322. G6PD deficiency may be accompanied by haemolysis if the patient

A takes a sulphonamide drug
B takes chloroquine
C eats French beans
D is a neonate
E takes penicillin

323. In pyruvate kinase deficiency

A inheritance is dominant with variable penetrance
B red cell potassium content is reduced
C clinical onset is usually at puberty
D splenectomy is beneficial
E survival to adulthood is common

324. In hereditary spherocytosis

A inheritance is X-linked recessive
B blood must be treated with sodium metabisulphite for the spherocytes to become recognisable
C haemolysis is extravascular
D splenectomy produces an effective cure
E splenectomy should be avoided in early childhood

325. Haemolysis is intravascular in

A   autoimmune haemolytic anaemia due to IgG autoantibodies
B   paroxysmal cold haemoglobinuria
C   microangiopathic haemolytic anaemia
D   march haemoglobinuria
E   paroxysmal nocturnal haemoglobinuria

326. In anaemia of chronic disorders it is usual to find

A   haemoglobin levels not below 9 g/dl
B   reduced serum iron
C   raised serum iron-binding capacity
D   increased iron in RE stores
E   increased red cell protoporphyrin

327. Recognised causes of macrocytosis include

A   alcoholism
B   chronic renal failure
C   hypothyroidism
D   aplastic anaemia
E   cytotoxic drug therapy

328. In the diagnosis of Addisonian pernicious anaemia

A   a raised MCV is not sufficient evidence of megaloblastic haemopoiesis
B   the serum folate level may be low
C   the RBC folate level is nearly always normal or raised
D   the serum B_{12} level is always reduced
E   neuropathy may occur before any morphological blood change

329. The following malignancies are particularly associated with severe manifestations of DIC:

A   mucin-secreting adenocarcinomas
B   renal carcinoma (hypernephroma)
C   metastatic prostatic carcinoma
D   acute promyelocytic leukaemia
E   small cell carcinoma of bronchus

330. Storage of blood causes predominant losses of

A fibrinogen
B factor VII
C factor VIII
D factor IX
E functional platelets

331. Graft versus host reactions following blood transfusion

A are mediated by transfused immunoglobulins
B occur only in immunocompromised subjects
C characteristically cause jaundice
D may occur in premature neonates
E may be prevented by prior irradiation of the transfused material

332. In platelet transfusion

A blood grouping can be ignored when using random-donor platelets
B frozen platelets are not immediately haemostatic
C platelets should be given to all patients with aplastic anaemia
D platelets should not be given to patients with disseminated intravascular coagulation
E it is important to assess the platelet count increment on each occasion

333. In the management of carbimazole-induced agranulocytosis

A serial neutrophil counts provide a valuable early warning of the onset
B withdrawal of the drug is usually followed by recovery
C corticosteroids have been clearly shown to hasten recovery
D antibiotics are of doubtful value
E leucocyte transfusions should be avoided because of the risk of immunisation

334. **Drug-induced thrombocytopenia**

    A may be caused by intravenous heparin
    B usually responds to withdrawal of the drug
    C is seldom improved by platelet transfusion
    D should not be treated with corticosteroids
    E has a better prognosis than drug-induced agranulocytosis

335. **Haemophilia A**

    A exhibits X-linked recessive inheritance
    B cannot occur in females
    C resulting in 10% Factor VIII activity or less is accompanied by
       severe manifestations
    D resulting in 25% Factor VIII activity or more may remain
       undiagnosed
    E causes prolongation of the thrombin clotting time

336. **In von Willebrand's disease**

    A inheritance is autosomal dominant
    B clinical consequences are severe in all cases
    C the bleeding time is prolonged
    D factor VIII levels may be reduced
    E the usual clinical presentation is a haemarthrosis

337. Schneider's first-rank symptoms of schizophrenia include

- **A** thought insertion
- **B** thought broadcasting
- **C** flattening of affect
- **D** poverty of speech
- **E** voices discussing the patient's thoughts or behaviour

338. The prognosis for the outcome of an episode of schizophrenia is relatively good if

- **A** there is no family history of schizophrenia
- **B** there is no obvious precipitating cause
- **C** the onset is gradual
- **D** there are prominent affective symptoms
- **E** initiative and drive are retained

339. In the management of schizophrenia, ECT is effective in relieving

- **A** catatonic symptoms
- **B** severe depressive symptoms
- **C** delusions
- **D** hallucinations
- **E** thought broadcasting

340. The following factors in a suicidal attempt suggest that the attempt was a serious one:

- **A** extensive premeditation (more than 3 hours)
- **B** telling others of the intention before the attempt
- **C** a suicide note
- **D** admitting suicidal intent
- **E** making a will beforehand

341. In Alzheimer's disease

- **A** amyloid plaques are found in the temporal lobes
- **B** a genetic component has been clearly shown
- **C** an infective cause has been clearly identified
- **D** there is a recognised association with dietary cadmium intake
- **E** treatment with cholinergic drugs has been shown to improve memory

342. Schizophrenia

A   is undoubtedly familial
B   is associated with cerebral atrophy
C   is benefited by dopaminergic drugs
D   occurs more commonly in subjects born during the summer months in the northern hemisphere
E   is associated with dominant hemisphere dysfunction

343. The following substances are recognised as cortical neuropeptides:

A   somatostatin
B   prostaglandin PGE_2
C   vasoactive intestinal polypeptide
D   cholecystokinin
E   substance P

344. In bereavement

A   sedatives are the main basis of therapy
B   grieving should be expected to begin within at least 2 weeks
C   stress-related conditions may be expected to improve
D   the death rate among bereaved persons is increased
E   suggestions by the bereaved of suicidal intentions may safely be ignored

345. Findings in pseudocyesis include

A   amenorrhoea
B   effacement of the navel
C   darkening of breast areolae
D   discharge from nipples
E   uterine enlargement

346. In puerperal psychosis

A   the onset is typically within the first 10 days after delivery
B   the patient is usually psychiatrically abnormal at the time of delivery
C   the patient is usually well-adjusted before pregnancy
D   delusions do not occur
E   affective features are extremely common

347. **Tricyclic antidepressants**

   A are best given in a single morning dose
   B should not be used in the presence of glaucoma
   C all cause sedation
   D are more likely to cause side-effects in the elderly
   E are safe when taken in overdose

348. **The following are correct statements:**

   A in sedating a violent patient, the drug of choice is haloperidol
   B severe confusion is best treated with a phenothiazine drug
   C stupor is usually due to organic illness
   D ECT is dangerous in depressive stupor
   E in panic attacks, somatic symptoms are usually due to hyperventilation

349. **In the periodic syndrome**

   A the onset of the pain is not related to meals
   B the symptoms always disappear before adulthood
   C the child is not kept awake at night
   D the finding of similar symptoms in another member of the family suggests that the diagnosis is wrong
   E drugs have no place in the treatment

350. **Enuresis**

   A is technically defined as failure to develop bladder control by the age of 3 years
   B is more common among boys than girls
   C is more common in the UK than in the USA
   D is more common in children of upper social class
   E can seldom be shown to be due to a single cause

351. **The following would favour a diagnosis of night terrors in a child rather than nightmares:**

   A total lack of awareness of surroundings in an attack
   B little or no amnesia for the episode
   C marked autonomic disturbance
   D association with REM sleep
   E screaming

352. **In the hyperkinetic syndrome**

    A   a history of brain injury is unusual
    B   abnormalities of the EEG have been described
    C   girls are more often affected than boys
    D   treatment with dexamphetamine is often beneficial
    E   tricyclic antidepressants should be avoided

353. **The following modes of therapy are appropriate for the clinical situations mentioned:**

    A   panic attacks: diazepam
    B   anxiety neurosis: amitriptyline
    C   phobic anxiety states: behaviour therapy
    D   anxiety neurosis: relaxation training
    E   palpitations: propranolol

354. **In the acute brain syndrome**

    A   hallucinations do not occur
    B   short-term memory is disturbed
    C   there is disorientation in time
    D   apathy may be a feature
    E   the mainstay of therapy is sedation with drugs

355. **Diagnostic criteria for anorexia nervosa include**

    A   weight loss of at least 15% of original body weight
    B   fear of becoming obese
    C   amenorrhoea
    D   disturbance of body image
    E   refusal to maintain weight above minimum normal for age and height

356. **Physical abnormalities which may be found in bulimia include**

    A   epileptic fits
    B   hoarse voice
    C   finger clubbing
    D   tetany
    E   enlargement of cervical lymph nodes

357. In bulimia nervosa

A   drugs should only be used as a last resort
B   cognitive behavioural therapy has been found effective
C   group therapy is completely ineffective
D   the prognosis is worse than for anorexia nervosa
E   vomiting is a recognised accompaniment

358. The drugs listed are drugs of first choice in the conditions mentioned

    A   complex partial seizures: clonazepam
    B   tonic-clonic (grand mal) seizures: carbamazepine
    C   absence seizures (petit mal): sodium valproate
    D   myoclonic seizures: ethosuximide
    E   secondarily generalised seizures: phenobarbitone

359. In the management of epilepsy, important interactions may occur between the following pairs of drugs:

    A   carbamazepine and warfarin
    B   ethosuximide and streptomycin
    C   phenobarbitone and oral contraceptives
    D   phenytoin and chloramphenicol
    E   sodium valproate and phenobarbitone

360. Measurement of serum drug levels is a useful guide to therapy with

    A   phenytoin
    B   carbamazepine
    C   phenobarbitone
    D   ethosuximide
    E   sodium valproate

361. In migrainous neuralgia

    A   men are more often affected than women
    B   a family history is almost invariable
    C   attacks occur at intervals of 1-2 weeks
    D   the pain is always unilateral
    E   ergotamine is often beneficial

362. In the management of a child who has had a first febrile convulsion

    A   hospital admission is desirable
    B   if the child is under 18 months of age, lumbar puncture is necessary
    C   the best emergency procedure is to give intramuscular diazepam
    D   if evidence of otitis media is found, antibiotic therapy should be started urgently
    E   no useful information can be obtained from an EEG

363. **After a first febrile convulsion, prophylactic anticonvulsant therapy is advisable if**

A   the first episode occurred at less than 1 year of age
B   there is a family history of febrile convulsions
C   the seizure was focal
D   the child is a male
E   a pre-existing neurological disorder was present

364. **The characteristic rhythms of the EEG have the following frequencies:**

A   α rhythm: 8-13 Hz
B   β rhythm: less than 4 Hz
C   δ rhythm: over 14 Hz
D   θ rhythm: 4-8 Hz
E   μ rhythm: 7-11 Hz

365. **The following muscle groups are supplied by the nerve specified:**

A   brachio-radialis: radial
B   triceps: radial
C   abductor pollicis brevis: ulnar
D   interossei: ulnar
E   tibialis anterior: sciatic (tibial branch)

366. **In deciding whether a cerebral vascular event is located in carotid or in vertebro-basilar territory, the following findings allow a definite distinction to be made:**

A   amaurosis fugax
B   dysarthria
C   dysphagia
D   facial paresis
E   hemi-sensory loss

367. **CT scan examination of a patient presenting with a stroke is desirable if**

   A   the patient is taking aspirin
   B   subarachnoid haemorrhage is a possibility
   C   cerebellar haemorrhage or infarction is a possibility
   D   the clinical diagnosis of stroke is doubtful
   E   vascular surgery is contemplated

368. **Intracranial tumours at the following sites are likely to produce the neurological changes mentioned:**

   A   frontal lesions: memory loss
   B   brain-stem tumours: damage to long motor and sensory tracts
   C   mid-line cerebellar tumours: inco-ordination of the limbs
   D   cerebellar hemisphere tumours: disturbances of gait
   E   cerebello-pontine angle tumours: impaired function of the Vth cranial nerve

369. **Complete surgical removal of an intracranial tumour should be seriously considered in the case of**

   A   meningioma
   B   glioblastoma multiforme
   C   cerebellar cystic astroctoma
   D   an accessible isolated metastasis
   E   temporal astrocytoma

370. **Radiotherapy plays an important part in the treatment of**

   A   meningioma
   B   posterior fossa medulloblastoma
   C   cerebellar cystic astrocytoma
   D   haemangioblastoma
   E   glioblastoma

371. **Early operation (within 48 hours) is preferable to delayed operation (2 weeks after haemorrhage) in the treatment of a bleeding intracranial aneurysm because**

   A   the post-operative mortality is lower
   B   recurrent bleeding is prevented
   C   cerebral ischaemia is less likely
   D   the overall mortality is lower
   E   it provides the opportunity of artificially raising the blood pressure if cerebral ischaemia does develop

372. **Idiopathic spasmodic torticollis**

   A   usually starts in childhood
   B   is painless
   C   leads to hypertrophy of the affected sternomastoid
   D   is nearly always persistent
   E   is resistant to all forms of treatment

373. **The diagnosis of brain death cannot be made if**

   A   one or both ankle jerks are present
   B   there is decerebrate posturing (extension of all four limbs)
   C   the jaw jerk is present
   D   the pupils are not widely dilated
   E   the cause of coma is unknown

374. **The following findings make the diagnosis of parkinsonism unlikely:**

   A   tremor confined to the head
   B   loss of weight
   C   oedema of the feet
   D   impaired ability to move eyes downward
   E   lack of blinking

375. **Characteristic findings in normal pressure hydrocephalus include**

   A   mental deterioration
   B   onset before puberty
   C   incontinence
   D   papilloedema
   E   enlargement of the ventricles

376. **In myasthenia gravis**

    A a thymoma is present in about 10% of patients
    B muscle weakness is nearly always accompanied by pain
    C ocular muscle involvement is nearly always asymmetrical
    D the tendon reflexes are greatly reduced or absent
    E removal of a thymoma causes remission of the symptoms

377. **A boy of 5 years of age is referred with a provisional diagnosis of Duchenne muscular dystrophy. The following findings would support the diagnosis:**

    A occurrence of DMD in a paternal uncle
    B intellectual retardation
    C asymmetrical distal myopathy
    D serum creatine kinase level of 20,000 IU/l
    E frequent painful muscle cramps

378. **In Kugelberg-Welander disease**

    A inheritance is autosomal recessive
    B death in the first 12 months is usual
    C the serum creatine kinase is grossly elevated (10-15,000 IU/l)
    D muscle biopsy shows a characteristic pattern
    E the carrier state can be identified with 95% certainty by gene analysis

379. **In motor neurone disease**

    A presentation is usually with wasting in the upper limbs and spasticity in the lower limbs
    B women are more often affected than men
    C the diagnosis should be confirmed by muscle biopsy
    D the diagnosis should be confirmed by EMG
    E a myelogram should always be performed

380. **The principal spinal root values are correctly assigned to these muscles**

    A   deltoid: C5
    B   triceps: C4
    C   small hand muscles: T1
    D   tibialis anterior: L2
    E   gastrocnemius: S1

381. **In carpal tunnel syndrome**

    A   abnormal signs are confined to the territory of the median nerve
    B   symptoms are referred to the hand only
    C   symptoms are aggravated by use of the hand
    D   the earliest sensory deficit is usually loss of temperature sensation
    E   surgical decompression produces immediate relief of pain

382. **In optic neuritis due to multiple sclerosis**

    A   the first symptom is always impairment of visual acuity
    B   complete unilateral blindness may occur
    C   the optic disc is usually swollen
    D   visual acuity usually begins to improve within 2-3 days
    E   persistent severe visual loss is rare

383. **There is now substantial evidence that the following mechanisms play a part in the genesis of multiple sclerosis:**

    A   genetic susceptibility
    B   persistent virus infection
    C   auto-immunity to myelin basic protein
    D   an environmental influence in childhood
    E   specific abnormality of lipid metabolism

384. **Recognised causes of dementia include**

    A   thiamine deficiency
    B   alcoholism
    C   hyperthyroidism
    D   Cushing's disease
    E   vitamin B_{12} deficiency

385. Atopic eczema in the infant characteristically affects the

    A cheeks
    B antecubital fossae
    C folds of the neck
    D groins
    E popliteal fossae

386. Lichen planus

    A causes intense itching
    B usually begins in childhood
    C produces depigmented lesions in coloured subjects
    D has a natural tendency to spontaneous remission
    E should not be treated with topical corticosteroids

387. Recognised causes of generalised pruritus include

    A pregnancy
    B hyperthyroidism
    C iron overload
    D drug abuse
    E aplastic anaemia

388. Fixed drug eruptions

    A usually involve multiple sites
    B often cause painful lesions
    C may be bullous
    D rarely involve the hands or feet
    E leave a hyperpigmented patch

389. The radiation involved in the following skin disorders is usually that known as UVA (320-400 nm):

    A sunburn
    B cutaneous lupus erythematosus
    C erythropoietic protoporphyria
    D photoallergic reactions
    E phototoxic rashes due to phenothiazine drugs

390. **The following disorders are clinically associated with vitiligo:**

    A Addison's disease
    B malignant melanoma
    C pernicious anaemia
    D acromegaly
    E diabetes mellitus

391. **The prognosis in malignant melanoma is worse if**

    A the lesion is more than 3.5 mm thick
    B the lesion is truncal in site
    C the patient is a female
    D the patient's age is less than 40
    E the lesion is ulcerated

392. **The following are characteristic features of generalised pustular psoriasis:**

    A fever
    B neutrophil leucocytosis
    C growth of *Staphylococcus aureus* on culture of the pustules
    D an invariably benign prognosis
    E good response to long-term treatment with prednisolone

393. **Rosacea**

    A is commoner in men than in women
    B may be improved by exposure to sunshine
    C will usually improve spontaneously within 6-10 weeks
    D responds to treatment with tetracycline
    E responds to treatment with topical corticosteroids

394. **Recognised causes of hirsutism (as opposed to hypertrichosis) include**

    A polycystic ovaries
    B congenital adrenal hyperplasia
    C porphyria
    D taking anabolic steroids
    E anorexia nervosa

395. **Leg ulcers due to arterial insufficiency**

    A   are usually sited over the medial malleolus
    B   are often surrounded by pigmented skin
    C   are very painful
    D   should be treated with strong elastic support
    E   should receive the same topical therapy as that suited to venous ulcers

396. **In the treatment of acne**

    A   dietary control is essential in all cases
    B   initial therapy in mild cases should include oral oxytetracycline
    C   topical benzoyl peroxide has both antimicrobial and keratolytic actions
    D   therapy can seldom be completed in less than 4 months
    E   13-cis-retinoic acid therapy should be reserved for the most severe cases

397. **In androgenetic baldness**

    A   occipital follicles are spared in men
    B   the commonest pattern in women is diffuse thinning
    C   some cases are precipitated by illness 2-3 months previously
    D   topical medication is of no avail
    E   cyproterone acetate may be valuable in men

398. **The following skin changes related to pregnancy always improve soon after delivery:**

    A   generalised pruritus
    B   spider naevi
    C   chloasma
    D   hirsutism
    E   telogen effluvium

399. **The following associations are correct:**

A   Beau's lines: arsenical poisoning
B   'half and half nails': chronic renal failure
C   clubbing of nails: tropical sprue
D   longitudinal white lines: Darier's disease
E   pitting of the nails: alopecia areata

400. **Erythema nodosum**

A   is more common in women than in men
B   does not involve the face
C   is painless
D   resolves without scarring
E   has no definable cause in 50% of cases

ANSWERS AND EXPLANATIONS

The correct answer options are given against each question. The references refer to Medicine International (2nd series); the figure in bold type indicates the issue numbers and the remaining figures are the page numbers.

1. **A B C**   **Ref:1,24**
Active immunisation is normally safe for children with protein-calorie-malnutrition. In very severe malnutrition it is best to give passive immunisation until the nutritional defect has been corrected, then move on to active immunisation. The results in developed countries have been spectacular; in developing countries there are problems arising from inadequate finance and administration to patients already immune.

2. **B D E**   **Ref:1,38,39**
Fansidar may safely be given with chloroquine and this combination may be necessary to give simultaneous protection against *Plasmodium vivax* and resistant strains of *P. falciparum*. Although Fansidar has not been officially cleared as safe in pregnancy, no case of teratogenicity has yet been reported and it should be given to pregnant women going to areas where chloroquine-resistant strains of *P. falciparum* are known to occur.

3. **A C D**   **Ref:1,10**
Children with fever and a cough are nearly always suffering from viral infections which resolve in a short time. Headache is another non-specific symptom common in minor infections in children.

4. **A B D**   **Ref:1,13:41,1725**
Renal haemangiopericytoma may cause abnormal secretion of renin, resulting in hypertension; cerebellar haemangioblastoma occasionally causes secondary polycythaemia.

5. **A B E**   **Ref:1,U1**
Vaccination against measles is recommended at 12-14 months or later, since maternal antibody can persist for up to 12 months.

6. **A B C E**   Ref:1,U5
A live attenuated vaccine is available against mumps and killed vaccines against rabies and pneumococcal infection. Active immunisation can be given against hepatitis B but not (at present) against hepatitis A.

7. **A D**   Ref:1,8
The incubation periods are: diphtheria, 2-5 days; mumps, 12-21 days; rubella, 14-21 days; scarlet fever, 1-3 days; malaria, 10-14 days.

8. **B C D**   Ref:1,29,30,32,33,34
The Paul-Bunnel test is negative in CMV infection and toxoplasmosis. In pregnancy, there is no risk to the fetus from the E-B virus but a definite risk from CMV (microcephaly, deafness, eye damage) and from toxoplasma (choroidoretinitis and severe neurological damage); it is therefore very important to establish an accurate diagnosis when a pregnant woman develops 'glandular fever'.

9. **A E**   Ref:2,48,51,45,43,48
Erythromycin is active against all serogroups of *Legionella pneumophila*. Clindamycin is a cause of pseudomembranous colitis since it stimulates growth of and toxin production by, *Clostridium difficile*; the correct drug is vancomycin. Mecillinam is active against many Gram-negative bacteria including *Salmonella spp.* and *Shigella spp.* but not against *P. aeruginosa*; gentamicin or tobramycin should be the first choice. The best choice for staphylococcal osteomyelitis would be clindamycin, fusidic acid or a penicillinase-resistant penicillin.

10. **A B D**   Ref:2,86,88
If the SAT is persistently negative, other tests may still demonstrate non-agglutinating IgG antibodies; these disappear after recovery so if they persist active infection is still present. IgM titres rise sharply in acute infections and exceed those of IgG or IgA.

11. **A B C D**   Ref:2,52,53,50
All the first four reactions are fairly commonly seen; aplastic anaemia occurs in less than 1 in 10,000 patients on sulphonamides.

12. **C D E**   Ref:2,64,65
Distinction must be made between *Salmonella* gastroenteritis, in which antibiotics are ineffective and the systemic forms of

salmonellosis, (typhoid and paratyphoid) in which antibiotic therapy is essential. *Shigella sonnei* usually produces only mild diarrhoea and antibiotics are unnecessary.

13. **B D E**   **Ref:2,76,77,78,79**
All three strains (gravis, mitis and intermedius) may cause severe disease. The smear appearances are unreliable; cultures from swabs from the nose or throat can be positively identified by an experienced observer within 15-20 hours. Neutralisation of toxin by antitoxin has an indirect antibacterial effect which checks the spread of the membrane.

14. **A B C**   **Ref:2,80,81,82,84**
The diagnosis is made on clinical grounds only. Autonomic instability, with abrupt changes in pulse rate and blood pressure, can occur in completely paralysed patients. An attack confers no immunity.

15. **B D E**   **Ref:2,69,70,71**
The organism is confined to man and there are no animal reservoirs. An attack does not always confer immunity.

16. **A E**   **Ref:2,74,75**
There is usually an absolute lymphocytosis and the ESR is normal unless broncho-pneumonia develops. Confirmation by culture of the organism is nearly always possible.

17. **A**   **Ref:3,105**
The reservoir in the Arctic is the fox population and in South America vampire bats. The domestic dog is the main vector in Europe but the reservoir is formed by foxes. In Asia the infection is perpetuated by carnivores both large and small - wolves, jackals, mongooses and civets.

18. **B E**   **Ref:3,93**
Paralysis is less common and less extensive in infants than in adults. Fatigue and physical exercise, once thought to play a part, are no longer believed to do so.

19. **B C E**   **Ref:3,125,126,128**
Common organisms are an important cause of infection. Acyclovir is ineffective against cytomegalovirus. *Pneumocystis* responds to

treatment with co-trimoxazole or pentamidine; the former is less toxic and is preferred.

20. **A C D E**   **Ref:3,131,132**
This condition, which is almost (though not entirely) confined to females, is also strongly associated with the use of vaginal tampons and is believed to be caused by toxins produced by *Staphylococcus aureus*.

21. **A C E**   **Ref:3,119**
The incubation period is up to 5 days in the cutaneous form. The regional lymph nodes are often enlarged and may provide a route for the extension of the disease to the blood stream.

22. **A D E**   **Ref:3,117**
Natamycin and nystatin are suitable for topical use only.

23. **B E**   **Ref:3,89,90**
Mumps is not notifiable in the UK. Meningitis is by no means rare but carries a good prognosis. Bilateral orchitis rarely causes sterility. Prednisone relieves the pain but does not alter the duration of orchitis or the risk of sterility.

24. **A B C D**   **Ref:3,97,98,99**
Idoxuridine and acyclovir may both be effective in different forms of HSV-1 infection.

25. **B C E**   **Ref:4,148,149,150**
Apart from some lymph node enlargement and the initial chancre (which it is impossible to identify with certainty) clinical examination is unhelpful and the diagnosis depends on clinical suspicion leading to blood examination. After the initial parasitaemia (about 5 days after infection) appearance of parasites in the blood is very irregular, hence the need for repeated sampling. Pentamidine is of doubtful value in rhodesiense infections: the drug of choice is suramin.

26. **B D**   **Ref:4,160,155,157,158**
Untreated espundia is usually fatal because of secondary infection. In visceral leishmaniasis the skin test does not become positive until after effective treatment; a positive test excludes active kala-azar. Pentamidine is a second-line drug in this condition; pentavalent antimonials should be used first.

27.   A C E   **Ref:4,**170
Rift Valley fever, Omsk haemorrhagic fever and yellow fever are the
only viral haemorrhagic fevers that can be prevented by vaccination.
Control of dengue fever depends mainly on mosquito eradication.
The vector of Lassa fever is unknown, but the animal reservoir is
thought to be in rodents; control measures should therefore aim at the
eradication of these and the prevention of contamination of human
food by their excreta.

28.   A C D   **Ref:4,**162,163
Louping ill and Crimean-Congo haemorrhagic fever are transmitted
by ticks.

29.   A D E   **Ref:4,**137,139,138
Amoebic dysentery is twice as common in men as in women and liver
abscess is seven times more common in men. The commonest sites for
ulcers are the caecum and the ascending colon. Massive haemorrhage
is very rare; the most dangerous complication is peritonitis. Emetine
compounds are the most potent amoebicides but also the most toxic;
in all but severe cases less toxic drugs should be used.

30.   C D E   **Ref:4,**179,180
A biphasic illness in Weil's disease is unusual. Jaundice appears on
day 4-6. Uveitis occurs in the first 6 months after the illness.

31.   C E   **Ref:4,**172,173,174,177
Tsutsugamushi disease is the original name for scrub typhus; it is a
disease of rural areas. The reservoir of infection is the mite
population; there is transovarial transmission from one mite
generation to the next, and uninfected mites are unable either to
acquire or to transmit the infection. The mites climb up to find a
warm, moist area of the body and bites are therefore commonest in
the groin, axillae and belt area.

32.   A C D E   **Ref:4,**133
Giardiasis occurs throughout the world but is commonest in the
tropics and subtropics. Peak prevalence is at about 10 years of age and
declines thereafter.

33.   A B C D E   **Ref:5,**205,201,204
All these filarial parasites are susceptible to treatment with
diethylcarbamazine. With some of them, notably *O. volvulus* and *Loa*

loa, the response to destruction of the parasites may be severe and reduced dosage or protection with corticosteroids may be necessary.

34. B C E   Ref:5,207,208
Most cases have some eosinophilia, but it may be transient. Cats are a less important source because they bury their faeces.

35. B C E   Ref:5,215,216,217,218
The skin lesions, which are few, contain very few bacilli. Enlargement of the ear lobes is characteristic of lepromatous leprosy. Dapsone resistance is now a world-wide problem and the WHO now recommends multi-drug regimes and bactericidal drugs for all forms of leprosy.

36. A D E   Ref:5,183,184,185,188,186
Infestation with *N. americanus* and with *S. stercoralis* is normally acquired through the penetration of larvae through the intact skin (usually of the feet and legs).

37. C E   Ref:5,219,220
The flea-bite usually causes no visible lesion but in an unusual form of the disease ('carbuncular plague') an ulcer develops at the site and this form has a good prognosis. The drug of choice is tetracycline, supplemented in seriously ill cases by streptomycin.

38. A E   Ref:5,190,191
Man acquires the infection by ingestion of eggs after contact with dogs. Only about 30% of cases develop an eosinophilia. The commonest site for cysts is the liver.

39. A D E   Ref:5,210,211,213
Abscess formation is not uncommon and the abscess may 'point' at unexpected sites, e.g. a psoas abscess in the groin. New bone formation is not commonly seen.

40. B D   Ref:5,196,198
Liver function tests only become abnormal in advanced liver disease; often the cause of abnormal results is hepatitis B virus. A nephrotic syndrome indicates amyloidosis or the deposition of immune complexes in the glomeruli. Metriphonate affects *S. haematobium* only; the drug of choice for *S. mansoni* is oxamniquine.

41. C E   **Ref:6,260,262**
Serum IgE is usually normal and the patients are not usually atopic. Investigations are essential; the diagnosis is one of exclusion and the investigations are necessary to rule out urticaria of known cause.

42. A B C E   **Ref:6,252**
Patients with AIDS show a profound T 'helper' cell lymphopenia.

43. A B D   **Ref:6,263**
Skin changes include urticaria or angio-oedema and cyanosis and/or pallor. Breathlessness may be due to laryngeal oedema or to an asthmatic attack.

44. A B D E   **Ref:6,227,228**
IgE has an affinity for mast cells and basophils but is secreted (like all immunoglobulins) by B-cells. The large molecular weight of IgM (900,000) hinders it from diffusing into interstitial fluid.

45. A B D   **Ref:6,232,229,230**
Acute anaphylaxis is an example of reaginic tissue damage. Drug-induced thrombocytopenia is an example of damage by membrane reactive antibody.

46. A B C D E   **Ref:6,235**
All are correct.

47. B C D E   **Ref:6,255,254,256**
Treatment of primary·vasomotor rhinitis is unsatisfactory and is directed mainly towards avoidance of the conditions which provoke symptoms. Oral antihistamines are of benefit in some cases; cromoglycate and systemic corticosteroids are ineffective.

48. A B D E   **Ref:6,242**
CH50 assay is only required if preliminary screening of C3 and C4 levels suggests a deficiency.

49. A C E   **Ref:7,286**
In determining the end-point of a trial, there should be an objective criterion and a single observer. Crossover design is a device whereby each patient serves as his own control, being tested with both active and placebo treatments.

50. **C D**   **Ref:7,271,272,273,274**
Many drugs, such as morphine, theophylline and phenytoin, have effects which are closely related to their plasma levels; prednisolone however shows a much less definite relation. In the case of overdosage with amitriptyline, most of the drug is outside the vascular compartment and cannot be removed by haemodialysis. After conjugation the larger molecules (MW>300) are excreted in the bile, the smaller in the urine.

51. **A B**   **Ref:7,297**
Cimetidine, metronidazole and chlorpromazine all <u>inhibit</u> hepatic mono-oxygenase activity.

52. **A B D E**   **Ref:7,311,312,313,314**
β_2 -agonists are less likely to produce β_1 -receptor-mediated cardiac side-effects. Inhaled salbutamol has an effect lasting for 3-4 hours; the only short-acting (1-2 hours) β_2 -agonist is rimiterol.

53. **A C D**   **Ref:7,302,303**
Measurement of drug levels is essential with procainamide but is of little value for ethosuximide and sodium valproate; the results bear little relation to the clinical effects.

54. **A D E**   **Ref:7,283**
Salbutamol is a β_2 -adreno-agonist. Disopyramide is a muscarinic antagonist. Labetalol is an adrenergic (α/β) antagonist. Apomorphine is a dopamine agonist. Clonidine is an α_2 -adreno-agonist.

55. **A B C E**   **Ref:7,292,291,290**
Cholestatic jaundice is more common in Scandinavian women taking oral contraceptives. Various HLA markers increase the risk of adverse reactions, especially to gold. Adverse reactions are more common in women than in men.

56. **A B C E**   **Ref:7,307**
Vitamin D is teratogenic in high dosage. Azathioprine is teratogenic in mice but no adverse effects on human fetuses have yet been recorded. Diethylstilboestrol if given during pregnancy predisposes to vaginal carcinoma in female children.

57. **A E**   **Ref:8**,323,324
These drugs reduce the coupling of excitation to contraction and so diminish the latter, i.e. negative inotropism. They are drugs of first choice in coronary artery spasm. They can be used, with caution, in conjunction with β-blockers, though the synergistic side-effects (cardiac failure, conduction defects) should be watched for carefully. In the case of verapamil, conduction defects are common and this drug should not be combined with β-blockers.

58. **C D E**   **Ref:8**,328,330,329,327
The loop diuretics (frusemide and bumetanide) should be reserved for patients with renal failure or resistant hypertension; bendrofluazide would be a better first choice. Prophylaxis against hypokalaemia is probably only necessary for those patients for whom it presents special risks - e.g. those on digoxin, with arrhythmias or with chronic liver disease; such patients should be given a potassium-sparing diuretic, not potassium supplements. Minoxidil may cause hirsutism. Atenolol and metoprolol are both β_1 -selective drugs.

59. **A B E**   **Ref:8**,336,337
Bismuth chelate heals peptic ulcers as effectively as cimetidine. The main side-effect of sucralfate is constipation.

60. **A C D E**   **Ref:8**,331,332
Warfarin acts by inhibiting the synthesis of prothrombin and factors VII, IX and X. It is not secreted in milk, but can cross the placenta freely, and its use is therefore not advisable during pregnancy except possibly during the second trimester.

61. **A B D**   **Ref:8**,350
Oral contraceptives cause a <u>rise</u> of some 30-70% in serum triglyceride and this may be related to the increased incidence of gall-bladder disease.

62. **A B C E**   **Ref:8**,356,355
Lithium is best used as a prophylactic, especially in bipolar affective illness. It crosses the placenta and is a well-recognised teratogen. It may make psoriasis and acne worse.

63. **A B**   **Ref:8**,321,320
Diplopia and ataxia may occur in patients taking high doses of carbamazepine and the use of divided doses, 3 or 4 times daily, may

give relief. Primidone is metabolized to phenobarbitone and the side-effects for the two drugs are identical. Gum hypertrophy is caused by phenytoin and not by sodium valproate.

64. **A B C E**   **Ref:8,**342,343,345,344
Chloroquine can cause retinal damage, the appearance of which may be difficult to distinguish from senile macular degeneration. Serum or plasma gold levels give little or no indication of either clinical efficacy or likelihood of side-effects.

65. **B C E**   **Ref:9,**374,376,377,375
Diazepam is a benzodiazepine and these drugs rarely cause serious effects in overdosage. Maprotiline and amoxapine are 'second generation' tricyclic antidepressants: symptoms of poisoning are similar to those of tricyclics generally and convulsions are common. Lithium overdosage may cause various CNS disturbances, including coma, but convulsions are uncommon.

66. **A B E**   **Ref:9,**364
The antidote for thallium poisoning is Prussian Blue and for iron poisoning, desferrioxamine.

67. **A B**   **Ref:9,**358,359,360,362
Plasma expansion is advisable for hypotension which does not respond to simple measures such as elevation of the foot of the bed. Skin bullae can result from poisoning by any CNS depressant. The usual background for self-poisoning is a personal or social problem: true psychiatric illness is relatively uncommon.

68. **B C D E**   **Ref:9,**380,381
Methylated spirit drinkers escape the toxic effects of the 5% of methanol in the liquid because the large amounts of ethanol monopolise the alcohol dehydrogenase and prevent conversion into formaldehyde and formate.

69. **A B D E**   **Ref:9,**369
Stimulation of the respiratory centre causes hyperventilation; uncoupling of oxidative phosphorylation causes accumulation of organic acids. Either hyponatraemia or hypernatraemia may occur; retention of sodium and water is usual, as is some degree of hypokalaemia.

70. C E   **Ref:9,396**
About half of all fatal reactions occur in subjects with no previous history of adverse reactions. Steroids and antihistamines may help in relieving urticaria, but the vital element of treatment in a severe case such as this is adrenaline.

71. A B E   **Ref:9,383,384**
Forced diuresis does not increase the excretion of digoxin (nor do haemodialysis, peritoneal dialysis or haemoperfusion). Gastric lavage should be performed if the patient is seen within 4 hours of taking the drug.

72. B D E   **Ref:9,389,388**
The effects are those of inhibition of cholinesterase activity at peripheral nerve endings, in the ganglia and the brain; hence meiosis, muscular flaccidity and weakness.

73. B D   **Ref:10,431,432**
With recessive inheritance, both parents are heterozygous for the abnormal gene and so will be two out of three of their children. In some conditions (retinitis pigmentosa, Duchenne muscular dystrophy) carriers can be detected by finding minor physical abnormalities.

74. A B C D E   **Ref:10,401,398**
All these conditions may be ANA-positive so the test is far from being specific for SLE. Up to 50% of patients taking hydralazine may show ANAs but only 10% develop lupus-like disease.

75. B D E   **Ref:10,436,426,429,431**
Triploidy implies the presence of 3 sets of 23 chromosomes, i.e. 69 in all. Down's syndrome is an example of trisomy; one pair of chromosomes is augmented to 3 (47 chromosomes in all). Mosaicism results from mitotic non-disjunction.

76. A D E   **Ref:10,430**
Cystic fibrosis and sickle-cell anaemia involve autosomal recessive inheritance.

77. A D E   **Ref:10,403**
Polyarteritis nodosa affects medium-sized arteries, polymyalgia rheumatica large and medium arteries.

78. **A C E**   Ref:10,405,406
Neurological involvement is very uncommon. The ESR is often normal.

79. **C D**   Ref:10,404
The condition is twice as common in women as in men. There may be marked constitutional disturbance with fever, weight loss and anaemia. Treatment should be cautiously withdrawn as soon as there is clinical relief and a fall in the ESR.

80. **B D**   Ref:10,401,400
Pregnancy is not contraindicated unless there is severe renal disease, but there is a risk of spontaneous abortion. Combined contraceptive pills often cause increased disease activity; the progestogen-only pill is safer. Renal biopsy can distinguish between focal proliferative, mesangial or membranous disease (potentially reversible) and diffuse proliferative disease (poor prognosis). The best index of disease activity is the level of antibodies to double-stranded DNA.

81. **B C D**   Ref:11,472,473
Probably toxic multinodular goitre evolves from a simple goitre which in some areas becomes autonomous. There is no evidence of increased TSH secretion. If treatment with antithyroid drugs is given, withdrawal of the drugs is followed by immediate relapse; the treatment of choice is with radioiodine, though as such goitres are relatively resistant to radiotherapy the dose needs to be large.

82. **B E**   Ref:11,475
Serum T4 may sometimes lie in the upper part of the normal range and the only way to exclude hyperthyroidism with certainty is to perform a TRH test. All β-blockers are effective in reducing the cardiac rate and this is an important item of treatment. Some 10% of patients with AF due to hyperthyroidism develop systemic embolism and anti-coagulants should be given unless there is some absolute contraindication.

83. **A B D**   Ref:11,475
Carbimazole is effective but has to be given by mouth; at present no intravenous preparation is available. Radioiodine acts too slowly to be of any help and in any case sometimes precipitates 'thyroid storm'.

84. **A B D E**   Ref:11,477
The effect of hypothyroidism on the menses is to cause menorrhagia.

85. A C D   **Ref:11,478**
The goitre is usually smooth and firm; occasionally it is hard enough to raise the suspicion of malignancy. About 75% of patients are euthyroid when first seen, but if the goitre is large T4 therapy may still be indicated, since this may reduce the size of the goitre.

86. A B C D E   **Ref:11,480**
Treatment should be started as soon as the diagnosis has been made clinically. The condition should be presumed to be due to pituitary or hypothalamic failure unless there is clinical evidence of primary thyroid failure.

87. A B   **Ref:11,441,442**
Males tend to present at a later age than females and often have the signs and symptoms of pituitary fossa expansion. The diagnostic level for serum prolactin is 2000 mIU/l.

88. A B E   **Ref:11,465,466,467**
In seriously ill patients the 'sick euthyroid' state may be confirmed by demonstrating a normal basal TSH level. Propranolol inhibits the de-iodination of T4 and so <u>reduces</u> T3 levels. Neonatal hypothyroidism has an incidence of about 1 per 4000 and can be detected by TSH estimation in capillary blood.

89. B   **Ref:12,525,527,526**
In a typical case the plasma potassium is less than 3.5 mmol/l, but 20% of all cases have levels of 3.5-4.2 mmol/l. The urinary potassium excretion is inappropriately <u>high</u>. The plasma levels of aldosterone and renin activity show a significant overlap with those found in essential hypertension. Adrenal hyperplasia is always bilateral and treatment should be with drugs, e.g. spironolactone.

90. A B C D E   **Ref:12,508**
In the presence of severe liver disease the contraindication is absolute; for the remainder it is relative.

91. B C D   **Ref:12,503**
The LH:FSH ratio is <u>increased</u>. Oestradiol levels are normal.

92. B C   **Ref:12,488,489**
Hypercalcaemia due to malignant disease often cannot be suppressed with corticosteroids. The serum phosphate level is not a good

discriminant. A serum PTH within the normal range but associated with hypercalcaemia may be 'inappropriately high' and consistent with the presence of a parathyroid adenoma.

93. **A C D**   Ref:12,500
Tamoxifen is an anti-oestrogen and danazol inhibits the release of pituitary FSH and LH; both tend to <u>reduce</u> oestrogen stimulation of breast tissue and have been used in the treatment of mild gynaecomastia. Cyproterone acetate is an anti-androgen and removes androgenic inhibition of oestrogen stimulation. Any cytotoxic drug, but particularly the alkylating agents, may damage testicular tissue and so reduce androgen levels. Tricyclic antidepressants, phenothiazines and some other drugs occasionally cause gynaecomastia by unknown mechanisms.

94. **A D E**   Ref:12,515
The amenorrhoea in anorexia nervosa is associated with a change in the pattern of LH secretion; prolactin levels are within the normal range and the same is true for ovarian failure, in which there is inadequate secretion of oestrogen, with high FSH levels. All the other conditions can cause high prolactin levels.

95. **B C D**   Ref:12,510,511,512
Testicular biopsy would only be necessary if semen analysis and hormone assays had been inconclusive. The woman's breasts should be examined to exclude galactorrhoea; if found, this would be highly suggestive of hyperprolactinaemia. A varicocele should be ligated - this will lead to pregnancy in about one third of such cases.

96. **A B C E**   Ref:12,493,494,496
The only use of bone age measurement is to define the proportion of growth which has already taken place and so to predict the maximum stature which can be attained. A child of short stature who is suffering from emotional deprivation has a normal GH response to pharmacological stimuli (e.g. insulin-induced hypoglycaemia) but commonly has a poor response to the physiological stimulus of sleep.

97. **A C D E**   Ref:13,552,553
The development of warmth and swelling in the foot of a diabetic is highly suggestive of a 'Charcot joint'. A bone scan will show new bone formation earlier than an X-ray and should be used to confirm the diagnosis.

98. **A C E** **Ref:13,**567,568
Good control of diabetes seems to reduce the incidence of macrosomia but unfortunately does not prevent it completely. When it is detected during pregnancy, mother and fetus must not be exposed to the risks of a full-term vaginal delivery. Either labour should be induced at 38 weeks or elective Caesarian section should be performed.

99. **A C E** **Ref:13,**564
Sexual maturation tends to be slightly delayed in diabetic children (especially in girls). There is no evidence of increased psychiatric morbidity. Microvascular disease is very uncommon in childhood but should never be ignored.

100. **A D** **Ref:13,**547,548
The circulating half-life of insulin is 4-5 minutes, so intravenous administration provides the flexibility needed in this urgent situation. Inappropriate administration of bicarbonate is dangerous; it should be given only on the basis of plasma pH readings and then only when the pH falls below 7.0. There is a substantial risk of venous and arterial thrombosis (especially in the elderly) and prophylactic anticoagulants may be indicated. Potassium should be given (20 mmol/hr IV) if the initial plasma level is below 6.0 mmol/l.

101. **B C D** **Ref:13,**533,534
Females predominate over males in Europe; the reverse is true in Japan and Malaya. Insulin levels are sometimes increased, due probably to hyperglycaemia or to decreased insulin sensitivity.

102. **A C E** **Ref:13,**554,555
Renal size is usually normal. There is a high incidence of all arterial disease and coronary artery disease is the commonest cause of death. Transplantation from a cadaver donor is much less satisfactory than from a live donor.

103. **A B D E** **Ref:13,**570,571
Fasting hypoglycaemia is precipitated by deprivation of food for a few hours or longer. Pyloroplasty and partial gastrectomy are causes of reactive post-prandial hypoglycaemia, in which symptoms occur 1 1/2 to 3 hours after a meal.

104. B D   **Ref:13,549**
Most sulphonylurea drugs can cause hypoglycaemia in therapeutic dosage and chlorpropamide is by no means the only offender; glibenclamide has frequently been responsible. The hypoglycaemia so caused is typically severe and prolonged and has a *higher* mortality than that due to insulin. Glucagon is best avoided because it causes insulin release as well as hepatic glycogenolysis.

105. B D E   **Ref:14,606,607,608**
Porphyrin synthesis is reduced by a high calorie intake and the treatment of acute porphyrias should include a carbohydrate intake of 1500-2000 kcal/24 hr. Morphine can safely be given. Venesection is recommended for cutaneous hepatic porphyria (a non-acute condition).

106. A B C   **Ref:14,582**
Familial hypertriglyceridaemia commonly causes eruptive xanthomata. In common hypercholesterolaemia xanthomata are not characteristically seen.

107. A C D E   **Ref:14,593,590**
There is failure of renal tubular reabsorption of bicarbonate, which causes acidosis (renal tubular acidosis).

108. B D E   **Ref:14,596,595**
The clinical features (including 'gargoylism') are very similar in the two conditions. In Hunter's disease a mild variant occurs with low or near normal intelligence and occasional survival to 30 years or more. All the mucopolysaccharidoses are transmitted by autosomal recessive inheritance, with the single exception of Hunter's disease (sex-linked recessive).

109. A C E   **Ref:14,617,618**
The serum alkaline phosphatase is usually normal or only slightly raised. Administration of vitamin D before removal of aluminium simply causes hypercalcaemia without clinical improvement. Given after aluminium removal it causes bone healing.

110. A B D   **Ref:14,620,621**
Serum calcitonin and PTH levels are usually normal. Disodium etidronate is usually given orally: absorption is poor and it should be given as a single dose in the middle of a 4-hour fast.

111. A C E   **Ref:14,623**
Osteogenesis imperfecta Type I is the common form, sometimes mild with osteoporosis only. Blue sclerae are seen in adult life. The deafness is due to abnormality or fracture of the auditory ossicles. Dentinogenesis imperfecta is more common in Type III but can occur in Type I.

112. B D E   **Ref:14,575**
An early adaptation to decreased protein intake is the increased utilisation of amino-acids for protein resynthesis, resulting in a sharp curtailment of nitrogen excretion. In severe undernutrition the cellular sodium pump activity is reduced, causing a loss of cell potassium and an increased entry of sodium into the cell; this leads to an increase in total body sodium even in the absence of oedema. Failure to synthesise the necessary metabolically active proteins leads to loss of zinc, copper and iron. Temperature regulation is impaired so that the patient is at risk from both hot and cold environments.

113. B C E   **Ref:15,649**
The serum uric acid level rises (hence the precipitation of acute gout in susceptible subjects) but this is due to decreased urinary excretion and not to increased production. The lactate:pyruvate ratio *increases* with a rise in the serum lactate level, which usually causes only trivial acidosis.

114. A D E   **Ref:15,651**
The serum ALT is not usually raised, whereas the AST usually is; an AST:ALT ratio of more than 2:1 is considered by some to be an indication of liver damage. The serum bilirubin is usually within normal limits.

115. C D E   **Ref:15,638**
Thiamine deficiency in non-drinkers, e.g. patients with hyperemesis gravidarum or gastric carcinoma, may cause Wernicke's encephalopathy. There may be confusion and ataxia only, or nystagmus may be present, without actual ophthalmoplegia.

116. A B D   **Ref:15,638**
The optic discs may become pale. The condition is at least partly reversible if tobacco and alcohol are withdrawn.

117. **A B C E**   **Ref:15,**631
The alcoholic condition resembles true Cushing's syndrome very
closely, with obesity, moon face, buffalo hump, striae and
hypertension; suppression of cortisol levels with dexamethasone is
incomplete.

118. **B C E**   **Ref:15,**631,632
Some two-thirds of alcoholics with macrocytosis have normoblastic
marrows. Iron should be given with caution since iron overload is
common among wine-drinkers.

119. **C D E**   **Ref:15,**632
The condition is characterised by acute onset of pain, swelling and
weakness of the affected muscles. Prominent U-waves in the ECG
indicate hypokalaemia, whereas in muscle damage potassium is
released and hyperkalaemia occurs.

120. **A C D E**   **Ref:15,**656
Low birth weight and reduced growth rate in the first year are usual.
All the other findings are recognised manifestations of the syndrome.

121. **A C**   **Ref:16,**667,668,669,670
A jerky pulse can also be caused by anxiety, severe mitral
regurgitation, and aortic regurgitation with severe heart failure. A
loud first heart sound, due to abrupt arrest of the mitral valve by the
chordae tendineae, can be produced in a normal heart beating at a fast
rate. Splitting of the second heart sound can often be detected in
normal subjects and may be caused by bundle branch block, right
ventricular overload and other conditions.

122. **A C D**   **Ref:16,**671
The severity of mitral stenosis is indicated by the *length* of the
murmur. The tricuspid murmur in ASD is very low-pitched.

123. **A C D**   **Ref:16,**675
In pressure overload (e.g. mitral stenosis, aortic stenosis) there is
myocardial hypertrophy and this causes little or no enlargement of the
outline of the chamber affected. In pericardial effusion the cardiac
silhouette is sharply defined because of diminished pulsation of the
borders.

124. **A B D E**   **Ref:16,689**
A high lung uptake in thallium scanning suggests raised left ventricular filling pressure.

125. **A D E**   **Ref:16,662**
The pain is characteristically relieved by sitting up and made worse by lying down. The traditional ECG finding of widespread raising of ST segments is actually uncommon and the ECG is rarely helpful. If the pericarditis is accompanied by formation of a pericardial effusion, the latter may be detected by echocardiography.

126. **A D**   **Ref:16,665**
Anginal pain is persistent and felt over periods of minutes rather than seconds. 'Non-specific' pain may radiate down the left arm but very seldom to the jaw and when relief comes from glyceryltrinitrate it is often only after 20-30 minutes. True anginal pain is facilitated by cold weather and often brought on by sexual intercourse.

127. **A C D**   **Ref:16,695,696**
In general, only valvular stenosis can be accurately measured by pressure measurements; regurgitation is best assessed by angiography. Pulmonary and tricuspid stenosis are measured by recording the pressures during withdrawal of the catheter from the pulmonary artery to the right atrium.

128. **A C**   **Ref:16,699,700**
The Fick principle requires the measurement of the A/V difference in oxygen content and therefore a simultaneous sample of mixed venous blood is also needed. In the thermodilution method the temperature of the blood in the pulmonary artery is recorded following the injection of saline at room temperature into the right atrium. Cardiac output at rest can be normal in quite severe heart disease and so is not a reliable indicator of early heart failure.

129. **A B D E**   **Ref:17,730**
Digitalis toxicity is a contraindication to the use of DC cardioversion.

130. **B**   **Ref:17,736,737**
The QRS complex is not markedly widened unless there is associated RBBB. Posterior fascicular block causes gross right axis deviation. BBB of all kinds remains stable in many patients. T-wave inversion in V1 is characteristic of RBBB.

131. **A C D E** Ref:17,714
ST segment depression over 4 mm would be a relative indication for stopping the test. All the other indications are absolute.

132. **A D E** Ref:17,703,704,706
Extrasystoles are particularly common in pregnancy. The normal limits of deviation of the cardiac axis are -30° to +90°. ST segment elevation is typical of cardiac infarction and can occur in the early stages without Q waves. T wave inversion in V2 and V3 can be a normal finding in negroes

133. **A D E** Ref:17,704,703
Hypertrophy of either ventricle is most surely diagnosed when findings additional to 'voltage changes', e.g. T wave inversion, are present. 'Voltage changes' alone may be seen occasionally in quite normal subjects, as may right or left bundle-branch block.

134. **D E** Ref:17,720
All of the first three findings have been reported in asymptomatic subjects and do not constitute firm indications for further action.

135. **A B C D E** Ref:17,701,702
All are correct.

136. **A B C D E** Ref:17,702
All are correct.

137. **A C D E** Ref:18,758,760,762
Polycythaemia of this order implies a serious risk of cerebral infarction. Surgery may be deferred, or may even be unnecessary, when the defect is of little haemodynamic significance.

138. **A B E** Ref:18,760,757,758
Frusemide promotes release of prostaglandins which will inhibit ductal closure; frusemide should not therefore be given when a persistent ductus is the main problem. In coarctation however re-opening the ductus may be beneficial by improving lower-segment perfusion. Diuretics are more important than digoxin in the treatment of neonatal cardiac failure. Morphine is beneficial in calming babies with heart failure or cyanotic attacks.

139.   B D E   **Ref:18,770,771,772**
Symptoms are seldom severe until the orifice has decreased to 1 cm²
or less. Digoxin may be given to patients in sinus rhythm to prevent
serious symptoms when AF develops. The key investigation is
echocardiography; catheterisation is only needed if there is doubt
about the severity of the stenosis or if an additional lesion is thought to
be present.

140.   A C D   **Ref:18,776,775**
There is always a systolic ejection murmur due to the increased stroke
volume. When symptoms develop, medical treatment has little to
offer unless heart failure has occurred; valve replacement is indicated.

141.   A B E   **Ref:18,752**
Aortic ejection clicks are caused by abnormal aortic valve cusps or a
dilated aorta. If the valve itself is normal no click is produced. In
severe pulmonary stenosis there is virtually no movement of the valve
and no click is heard.

142.   A C E   **Ref:18,753**
Innocent murmurs may vary with change in posture. The venous hum
is continuous.

143.   A B   **Ref:18,777,780**
Valve repair should be attempted first in mitral regurgitation; if the
repaired valve is still incompetent, the operation continues with valve
replacement. Grafted valves deteriorate more quickly in younger
patients, and the risk of thromboembolism is higher with mitral than
with aortic valve replacement.

144.   A C E   **Ref:18,767,768**
The systolic murmur of mild mitral incompetence may persist
throughout life unaccompanied by any cardiac disability. Almost all
patients with rheumatic heart disease have involvement of the mitral
valve.

145.   A E   **Ref:19,781,782**
Mean pressures for Bahamians (both male and female) fall into the
'hypertension' limits defined by the WHO criteria and the means for
north-eastern Japanese into the 'borderline hypertension' limits.

146. **A B C**   **Ref:19,789,788,790**
Extreme exertion (e.g. a marathon run) may cause the production of granular, and occasionally erythrocyte, casts in normal subjects. Polycystic kidneys can nearly always be detected by clinical examination.

147. **A C E**   **Ref:19,792,793**
Malignant hypertension is not an indication per se for parenteral therapy as sudden reduction in blood pressure carries a risk of cerebral infarction. Labetalol should be avoided in LV failure; it is a combined α- and β-adrenergic blocker and the latter activity will make the LV failure worse. Diazoxide causes tachycardia which has been associated with ECG abnormalities in patients with IHD.

148. **A**   **Ref:19,803**
See Table 8 of the article by Professor Mitchell.

149. **B E**   **Ref:19,804,805**
The clinical findings are non-specific; of all patients with suggestive symptoms and signs only about half can be shown to have thrombosis on full investigation. Impedance plethysmography gives false-positive results in several disorders, including cardiac failure and hypotension. Doppler ultrasound is relatively insensitive to calf vein thrombosis.

150. **D E**   **Ref:19,810,811**
Heparin is best given by continuous intravenous infusion with repeated monitoring of the PTT; intermittent injection carries a higher risk of bleeding. Heparin should be continued for *5 days* after starting warfarin, since this time is required for the full antithrombotic effect to be produced. There is now clear evidence that long-term warfarin therapy significantly reduces the risk of recurrent venous thromboembolism.

151. **A D E**   **Ref:19,813,814,816**
Patients with pulmonary sarcoid or systemic sclerosis who develop cor pulmonale have a very bad prognosis. Long-term oxygen therapy has been shown to be of definite benefit when the cause is obstructive airways disease, but the expense means that relatively few patients can be given this treatment. Vasodilators act on the systemic as well as on the pulmonary vessels and if they are given in primary pulmonary hypertension they may cause systemic hypotension.

152.   E   Ref:19,818,819
Items A and B are typical of Buerger's disease. The condition was at one time thought to be commoner in Jews but it is certainly not confined to the Jewish race and may well be seen in non-Jewish subjects. Smoking exacerbates the condition but is not its cause. The arteries mainly affected are those below the politeal and it would be unusual for both femoral pulses to be obliterated.

153.   A C D   Ref:20,826
See opening paragraphs of article by Professor Shaper.

154.   A C D E   Ref:20,839,840
Sublingual glyceryl trinitrate has a duration of action of about 30 minutes, compared with about 1 hour for isosorbide dinitrate. Proof of adequate β-blocker dosage depends on the demonstration that *exercise* tachycardia is reduced; bradycardia at rest is insufficient evidence.

155.   A C E   Ref:20,841
A β-blocker should be prescribed immediately, provided there is no contraindication (e.g. heart failure or bronchospasm). The patient can use his supply of sublingual nitrates to deal with a sudden attack of pain. Intravenous nitrate therapy is safe provided the blood pressure is measured at frequent intervals.

156.   All false   Ref:20,842,843
There is evidence that intravenous streptokinase can restore flow in a blocked coronary artery, but no firm agreement that this is accompanied by reduction in mortality or improvement in ventricular performance.

157.   A D E   Ref:20,843,844,845
The R on T extrasystole is a warning of threatened ventricular fibrillation and prophylaxis is essential. Other ventricular extrasystoles, even in runs of up to 12 beats, are not warnings of VF and may be ignored. Atrial fibrillation is always transitory and usually needs no treatment; if causing a very fast ventricular rate and/or cardiac failure, it may be treated with amiodarone. Cardioversion is rarely successful and even if it is may be followed by recurrence.

158.   A   Ref:20,849,850
There may be good reason, on various grounds, for introducing items

B to E, but none of them has been shown clearly to reduce the risk of subsequent infarction. The results for stopping smoking are, however, unequivocal.

159.   A B E   **Ref:20,**836
Anterior infarction and tachycardia on admission are associated with high mortality in hospital.

160.   A B C D E   **Ref:20,**837
All the items yield useful information.

161.   A B C   **Ref:21,**892
Cholestyramine and rifampicin *reduce* the effect of warfarin and the dose would need to be increased.

162.   B C   **Ref:21,**872,873
Maximum vulnerability occurs with a regurgitant stream and a large pressure drop across a small orifice, e.g. *mild* aortic or mitral regurgitation or a *small* VSD. The incidence in developed countries appears to be increasing. Only about 50% of patients have previously known heart disease.

163.   A B D E   **Ref:21,**873,874,875
The complement level is only reduced in the presence of nephritis, so this is a useful diagnostic investigation. Renal involvement is usually a focal proliferative nephritis but occasionally the lesion is diffuse with impairment of renal function. The threat of embolism and of rapid destruction of valves means that treatment must be delayed only long enough to allow blood cultures to be taken.

164.   A B   **Ref:21,**876
The vegetations are large and friable and there is a serious risk of embolism. Blood cultures are often negative because fungaemia is usually intermittent. Surgical excision of the affected area is nearly always necessary to effect a cure.

165.   A B E   **Ref:21,**871
The effect of vasodilators in patients with cardiac failure is different from that in normal subjects; the reduction in blood pressure is dominant and cardiac output increases despite the fall in ventricular filling pressure. Improvements in haemodynamics are not a good guide to the degree of symptomatic relief.

166. **A B D E**   **Ref:21,865**
The normal or raised blood pressure is an important distinction from myocardial infarction. Cardiac enzymes are often raised and so may be misleading.

167. **A B**   **Ref:21,886,887**
Usually, removal of 20% of the effusion is sufficient. The ventricles are *underloaded* hence the dangerous fall in cardiac output.

168. **A D E**   **Ref:21,888**
The spleen may be enlarged and this observation would not be inconsistent with the diagnosis. There are usually no murmurs.

169. **All false**   **Ref:22,906,909,910**
All the findings mentioned can occur in rheumatoid arthritis. Many patients have carpal tunnel syndrome due to the swelling at the wrist. Episcleritis is common. Echocardiography reveals significant pericardial effusion in many cases but the risk of tamponade is very small. Splenomegaly is found in 5% of cases and generalised lymphadenopathy in about 50%.

170. **A C D E**   **Ref:22,910**
DNA binding is not elevated.

171. **B C D E**   **Ref:22,920,919**
Juxta-articular osteoporosis is characteristic of rheumatoid arthritis and is an important diagnostic feature when confusion arises between the two conditions.

172. **A E**   **Ref:22,901**
Gram-staining and microscopy of the aspirate will show the presence of pus cells and organisms and will thus confirm the diagnosis, but knowledge of the antibiotic sensitivities of the infecting organism is needed for the most effective treatment to be devised. Culture of the aspirate may be negative if the infecting agent is the gonococcus. Repeated aspiration usually provides sufficient drainage, except in inaccessible joints such as the hip.

173. **A B C E**   **Ref:22,904**
The pupil is usually small and may be irregular if there have been previous attacks. Hypopyon is a visible collection of pus cells in the anterior chamber.

174. B C D E   **Ref:22,**913,912,917
The incidence of HLA-B27 in white subjects is 6-14%.

175. A C D E   **Ref:22,**923
Subcutaneous nodules are common over pressure points, especially
the olecranon. Active disease persisting into adult life causes serious
disability in 25%.

176. C D   **Ref:22,**924
The diagnosis is made clinically from the fever, rash,
lymphadenopathy and hepatosplenomegaly. There are no specific
laboratory tests. Leucocytosis may exceed 40×10^9 /l. The fever is
characteristically remittent, being high in the evening and normal the
next morning.

177. A B C   **Ref:23,**938
Mefenamic acid belongs to the fenamic acid group and diclofenac to
the phenylacetic acid group.

178. A   **Ref:23,**966,967,968
Only in rheumatoid arthritis is there a high incidence (75%) of
remission during pregnancy. In SLE improvement occurs in about
one third of the patients. In ankylosing spondylitis the proportion is
some 10-20%; in systemic sclerosis there is no effect and in
dermatomyositis there is usually deterioration.

179. A B D E   **Ref:23,**959,960
A fall in plasma urate from a previously high level can precipitate
acute gout, e.g. following administration of salicylates.

180. B D E   **Ref:23,**942
A total dose of 1000 mg should be given before abandoning the
treatment on the ground of no response. A trace of protein only
implies a need for caution, but urine monitoring must be maintained
scrupulously.

181. A B D   **Ref:23,**943
The patient with loss of taste sense should be reassured and told that
this will recover even if the drug is continued. Nausea and vomiting
may require temporary reduction of the dose, but only rarely a
complete withdrawal.

182. **A B C E** Ref:23,970
Shigella flexneri and *S. dysenteriae* can both cause arthritis, but not *S. sonnei.*

183. **A C E** Ref:23,970
There are no destructive changes and no long-term effects. Local corticosteroid injection is an accepted form of treatment.

184. **A B D E** Ref:23,965
The skin eruption (when present) resembles cellulitis or erysipelas, occurring over one or other leg below the knee.

185. **A C** Ref:24,1005
The blood group carrying an increased risk is A. Consumption of dairy produce and fresh vegetables has a *negative* relationship with gastric cancer.

186. **B C D** Ref:24,1006,1007
ACG also causes IM, of which the incompletely differentiated type is strongly related to gastric cancer. Completely differentiated IM, producing mucosa resembling that of the small intestine, is not strongly related to gastric cancer.

187. **A C D E** Ref:24,987
Hypokalaemia causes constipation. Chagas' disease (American trypanosomiasis) can cause parasympathetic denervation of oesophagus and/or colon, in the latter case producing a form of megacolon.

188. **C D E** Ref:24,974,975
Some patients feel the sensation only in the throat and it can radiate to the back. It may be the predominant symptom in peptic ulceration and may occur if neutral or alkaline gastric juice containing bile undergoes reflux.

189. **B D E** Ref:24,979,978
Morning nausea and inability to eat for some hours after vomiting are both common symptoms in non-organic dyspepsia. Early satiety and loss of weight would be suggestive of gastric cancer and painless diarrhoea of alcohol abuse.

190. **C E**   **Ref:24,**1000,1002
Gastric acid production in patients with gastric ulcer is normal or reduced (much increased in duodenal ulcer). GU is commoner in patients of lower socio-economic class. Dosage of cimetidine or ranitidine should be spaced out (e.g. b.d. or t.d.s.), but single bedtime doses are satisfactory for duodenal ulcer.

191. **B C E**   **Ref:24,**986,985
The measured osmolality exceeds the amount of (Na + K) x 2 by more than 50 mmol/l. This osmotic gap is commonly a disaccharide, the commonest being lactose (in lactase deficiency) but if the patient is taking an osmotic purgative, e.g. magnesium sulphate, the same gap will appear.

192. **C**   **Ref:24,**992,993
About 35% of patients with pain due to reflux have no demonstrable abnormality of the oesophagus. Reflux is commonly associated with sliding hiatus hernia but only rarely with the rolling variety. Cimetidine treatment produces symptomatic relief but has little effect on established oesophagitis. Surgery is usually effective and is the treatment of choice when the symptoms are severe and the patient is fit enough.

193. **B C**   **Ref:25,**1013,1014,1015,1016
The mortality remains at about 10%, mainly because of the rising proportion of elderly patients. Bed rest is clearly necessary in the presence of hypovolaemia but otherwise it is not indicated. H_2-receptor antagonists may possibly help to prevent re-bleeding but there is no evidence that they stop bleeding.

194. **A B C**   **Ref:25,**1044,1045
The molecules of IgA are joined together by a small peptide (the J chain) and this dimer binds to a glycopeptide (the secretory piece); the latter provides protection against proteases. Complement is not involved and interaction of antigen and secretory IgA does not cause tissue injury. Antigen absorption is reduced or prevented.

195. **A C D E**   **Ref:25,**1045,1046
Symptoms caused by immunological mechanisms (usually mediated by IgE) after the ingestion of food are defined as food allergy. However urticaria and asthma can occur in food intolerance and complement is activated by the alternative pathway.

196. **A D E**   Ref:25,1028,1029
The disease is also found in South Africa. Abdominal pain may occur. In treatment, broad spectrum antibiotics, radiotherapy and chemotherapy may be helpful.

197. **B C D E**   Ref:25,1027,1028
Constipation does *not* rule out the diagnosis. In children transient mucosal damage from other causes (e.g. viral enteritis) is common and the diagnosis is not certain until a histological relapse after challenge has been confirmed.

198. **A D E**   Ref:25,1039,1036,1037
Excess carbohydrate calories are stored as fat in the liver. When intravenous fat is given the glucose input must be *reduced* below the metabolic requirement for energy, otherwise the high insulin levels will reduce the oxidation of fat and hyperlipidaemia will result.

199. **A B D E**   Ref:25,1019
Rectal bleeding should not be accepted as due to IBS and should always alert the physician to an organic cause. Loss of weight can occur but is usually of a few pounds only and associated with anorexia.

200. **A C**   Ref:25,1042,1043
When the diarrhoea is severe it causes hypokalaemia and acidosis. The fasting VIP level is always greatly raised. 90% of cases show a response to streptozotocin.

201. **A D**   Ref:26,1078
A 1-cm sigmoidoscope gives an adequate view and causes less discomfort than wider instruments. Biopsies are usually taken below the level of peritoneal reflection and perforation will therefore usually resolve with conservative treatment. There are no contraindications to proctoscopy or sigmoidoscopy. In painful conditions of the anus, rectal examination can be made possible by the use of a local anaesthetic.

202. **A B D E**   Ref:26,1081,1082
If diverticular disease is present or suspected, this does not constitute an adequate explanation for trivial bleeding and another cause must be sought; very rarely it may cause torrential bleeding.

203.   A C E   **Ref:26,1057**
The presence of granulomas and of widespread sub-mucosal inflammation would point strongly to Crohn's disease.

204.   B C D   **Ref:26,1062,1060**
There is a very good chance that a female patient in remission who becomes pregnant will remain in remission throughout gestation. Broad spectrum antibiotics should be *avoided* as they may precipitate a relapse.

205.   B C D   **Ref:26,1068,1069**
About a third of all patients over 65 can be shown by barium enema to have colonic diverticula and most of these patients have no symptoms. The diagnosis of diverticulitis therefore depends on the clinical findings more than on the X-ray. Morphine should be avoided because it increases muscle spasm and can precipitate perforation. Metronidazole is a safe and effective treatment.

206.   C D E   **Ref:26,1069,1070**
The two drugs most likely to cause colitis are lincomycin and clindamycin. The risk of developing colitis is unrelated to the dose, route of administration or length of the treatment course. The diagnosis is confirmed by the demonstration in the stool of the toxin of *Clostridium difficile*.

207.   A C D E   **Ref:26,1050,1051**
The skin condition associated with Crohn's disease is erythema nodosum. Erythema annulare centrifugum has no connection with it.

208.   A C   **Ref:26,1055**
Recurrences are frequent and are commoner than in adult patients. Corticosteroids are essential in many cases; if given on alternate days the stunting effect on growth is minimised and the control of the disease may in fact promote growth. Growth is particularly retarded in the presence of strictures and surgery to relieve these must be performed before epiphyseal closure if stunting is to be prevented.

209.   A   **Ref:27,1109**
The vitamins whose absorption is impaired are the fat-soluble group (A and D). Absorption of vitamin B_{12} is not normal but clinical evidence of insufficiency is rare.

210. **B C D**   **Ref:27,1110,1111,1113**
Men are more commonly affected. Neither chemotherapy nor radiotherapy have any place in treatment; they are ineffective and both involve high morbidity.

211. **A C D E**   **Ref:27,1107**
Acute pancreatitis may be caused by a *rise* in serum calcium level; it may also itself *cause* a secondary *fall* in calcium level.

212. **A C D E**   **Ref:27,1114,1115**
The pancreas exhibits impaired *secretion* of bicarbonate; the lowered osmotic pressure of the pancreatic juice allows increased absorption of water, which in turn leads to high protein concentration and blockage of ducts by precipitated protein.

213. **A C D E**   **Ref:27,1116**
Babies placed in too warm an environment lose large quantities of chloride; the renal conservation of chloride leads to potassium loss and hypokalaemic *alkalosis*.

214. **C E**   **Ref:27,1128**
The disease may begin at any time from early childhood until middle age. Permanent joint damage is uncommon. Jewish patients are particularly likely to develop amyloidosis.

215. **A E**   **Ref:27,1123**
Any part of the gut may be involved, but particularly the stomach and small intestine. The usual presentation is either with malabsorption or with obstruction. If no specific cause (e.g. food sensitivity or infestation with gut parasites) can be found, corticosteroids often cause improvement.

216. **A D**   **Ref:27,1118,1119,1120**
Rectal gonorrhoea can be confirmed by rectal Gram-stained smear examination in only about 50% of cases. LGV should be treated with oxytetracycline. Non-A non-B hepatitis is relatively uncommon in homosexuals; those chiefly at risk are drug addicts and haemophiliacs. The usual cause of death in Kaposi's sarcoma is opportunistic infection.

217. **B E**   **Ref:28,1147**
Mucoceles are the result of injury to salivary gland ducts. They usually

develop rapidly and sometimes last for only a few hours. Incision and drainage may be followed by recurrence; the correct procedure is excision.

218. **A D E**   Ref:28,1147,1148
The disease is chronic but usually reaches a 'plateau' and does not progress further. In about 1% of patients the lymphoid infiltration of the glands progresses through lympho-proliferation to non-Hodgkin's lymphoma.

219. **B C**   Ref:28,1153
The key is the gross elevation of ALT which indicates active damage to hepatic cells (absent in A, D and E).

220. **B D**   Ref:28,1181
The virus has still not been identified. The incubation period is 6 to 8 weeks. The disease is anicteric in 50% of patients, but up to 25% may develop cirrhosis.

221. **A D E**   Ref:28,1163
Hepatitis A virus may occasionally be shed during this period. Bed rest is unnecessary and choice of diet may be left to the patient.

222. **A C**   Ref:28,1165,1166
Hepatitis A is the second commonest cause (after hepatitis non-A, non-B). Serum transaminases commonly fall as the patient's condition deteriorates. The early acid base disturbance is either respiratory alkalosis, due to hyperventilation, or metabolic alkalosis with hypokalaemia.

223. **A B C D E**   Ref:28,1142,1143,1144
All are true associations.

224. **C D**   Ref:28,1134,1135
There is no evidence of an autoimmune basis. About one third of all patients have a positive family history, but there is no regular Mendelian inheritance and only weak HLA associations. Some 70-80% of sufferers are non-smokers and giving up smoking may precipitate the first attack.

225. **A C**   Ref:29,1181
The transaminase levels are raised to 2-5 times the upper limit of

normal. Serum immunoglobulin levels are normal. In some patients in whom the cause is hepatitis B there may be evidence of active viral replication (HBeAG positive) and these may progress to cirrhosis over many years; these patients may be benefited by antiviral therapy.

226. A B D E   **Ref:29,**1182
Half the patients have some other autoimmune disorder.

227. B D E   **Ref:29,**1171,1173,1172
The investigation of choice in suspected acute cholecystitis is ultrasonography. Liver tumours contain no Kuppfer cells and so fail to concentrate labelled colloid.

228. B D   **Ref:29,**1189,1190
The histological changes may be very patchy and a single biopsy is often only 'consistent with' PBC rather than 'diagnostic'. There is no effective treatment; immunosuppressive drugs have no effect on survival. Corticosteroids given over long periods may promote osteoporosis, which is the main bone disorder; osteomalacia is much less common than was previously thought.

229. A B D   **Ref:29,**1193,1194,1195,1196
Vasopressin and glypressin are both coronary artery vasoconstrictors, so any ECG evidence of myocardial ischaemia would be a contraindication to their use. The oesophageal balloon must not be inflated for longer than 24 hours otherwise oesophageal ulceration may occur. Propranolol is a valuable agent for reducing portal venous pressure in long-term management.

230. B C D   **Ref:29,**1201,1202,1203
The common presenting symptoms of hepatocellular carcinoma are pain, weakness, anorexia and weight loss and abdominal swelling; jaundice is relatively uncommon. The commonest benign hepatic tumour is cavernous haemangioma.

231. A C D   **Ref:29,**1186,1187
There is no such enzyme as ferritin transferase and in fact the basic functional defect responsible is unknown. The definitive test is the hepatic iron concentration as measured on a biopsy sample. Once the diagnosis is made life-long therapy and surveillance are required.

232. **A C** Ref:29,1190,1191,1192
A low-fibre diet is thought to predispose to gallstones. 10-30% of all stones are radio-opaque. Medical therapy with chenodeoxycholic acid or ursodeoxycholic acid is effective in more than 50% of patients with cholesterol stones and a functioning gall-bladder.

233. **B C E** Ref:30,1251
Onset is sudden, with fever, sweats, arthralgia, sore throat and diarrhoea. Lymphopenia and thrombocytopenia are usual. Suppressor T cells are increased but the number of T helper cells is unchanged.

234. **A B D E** Ref:30,1253
The gastrointestinal tract is nearly always involved. There is a higher prevalence of HLA-DR5 in these patients than in the general population.

235. **A B E** Ref:30,1250
Infections with *Cryptococcus* and *Histoplasma* are rare in UK patients with AIDS.

236. **B D** Ref:30,1242,1243,1244,1245
Recovery from persistent generalised lymphadenopathy (PGL) is well documented. Sero-conversion many months or even years after infection has been reported. Nearly all patients with PGL are sero-positive but occasionally sero-conversion occurs *after* its clinical development. About 65% of babies born to infected mothers become infected and of these about half may be expected to develop AIDS within 2 years.

237. **A C D E** Ref:30,1248,1249
AIDS causes activation of B cells with resulting *increase* in serum gamma-globulin but the response to new antigens is impaired. Hence the susceptibility of AIDS patients to intercurrent infections; serological diagnosis of the infection also becomes unreliable and isolation of the organism, or histology, is preferred.

238. **A B D** Ref:30,1233,1234
The first attack is usually relatively severe and recurrences milder. Acyclovir is effective in shortening the attack.

239. A   **Ref:30,1223,1225**
Smear examination from male urethral pus is accurate in at least 95%
of cases. The remaining sites are complicated by the presence of other
organisms which may be mistaken for *Neisseria gonorrhoeae* and
culture is needed for certain identification.

240. C D E   **Ref:30,1219**
The rash starts on the trunk and the proximal segments of the limbs;
the palms and soles are *not* spared.

241. A B D E   **Ref:31,1259,1260**
Falsely high levels are found after prolonged fasting and in severe
hyperglycaemia (interference by ketone bodies and unidentified
substances respectively).

242. A D   **Ref:31,1257**
The upper normal limit of plasma osmolality is 295 mOsmol/kg. The
calcium figure given would be normal for *total* serum calcium; the
ionized fraction is normally about half the total. Serum inorganic
phosphate has an upper normal limit of about 1.6 mmol/l.

243. A D   **Ref:31,1294,1295,1296**
Pre-eclampsia does not usually recur; hypertension due to underlying
renal disease usually recurs in all subsequent pregnancies. Lupus
nephritis responds well to treatment. Polycystic disease may be
accompanied by renal tract infection and may deteriorate rapidly
during pregnancy.

244. A D E   **Ref:31,1266,1267,1268,1269**
Results from low-osmolar media are comparable to those from
conventional agents. Calculi composed of xanthine, uric acid and
cystine all have a high density in CT scanning.

245. A B C E   **Ref:31,1276,1277,1279**
Low back pain is almost never the result of renal disease. Cloudiness
of the urine without other symptoms is usually due to phosphate
precipitation.

246. A C D E   **Ref:31,1283**
Enuresis is more common in first-born children.

247.   B C   Ref:31,1286,1285
Most children over 7 can be taught to use the alarm, some as young as 6. The alarm should be placed out of reach of the child, so that he/she has to get out of bed to switch it off. The usual cause of alarm failure is accidental or deliberate switching off by the child on getting into bed.

248.   A B C D E   Ref:31,1288,1289
All are true. Radiotherapy involving irradiation of the bladder may cause fibrosis of the bladder wall and loss of normal visco-elasticity. Autonomic neuropathy due to diabetes or other causes may cause loss of bladder sensation.

249.   B C E   Ref:32,1298
The usual upper normal limit for 24-hour proteinuria is 200 mg. Orthostatic proteinuria may accompany glomerular disease and is not necessarily benign.

250.   A B E   Ref:32,1303,1302
The deposits in Berger's disease and in Henoch-Schönlein nephritis consist of IgA.

251.   A B D E   Ref:32,1316
Patients with non-oliguric ARF have a relatively low mortality (10-40%). The other factors carry a mortality of 80-90%.

252.   A B D   Ref:32,1320
A rise in serum alkaline phosphatase (over 130 IU/l) is the earliest change. Vitamin D has been superseded in this situation by 1-α-hydroxycholecalciferol or 1,25,-dihydroxycholecalciferol, since these have shorter biological half-lives and allow more flexible management.

253.   A C   Ref:32,1322,1323,1324
Dietary restriction is needed for most patients, involving control of protein and potassium intake and possibly of sodium, water, phosphate and saturated fat. Most patients are not iron-deficient and blood transfusion has a beneficial immunological effect on subsequent transplantation.

254.   A B C E   Ref:32,1326
In some patients with pre-existing hyperlipidaemia, CAPD makes this worse if large volumes of high osmolar fluid are used.

255. **B E** Ref:32,1329,1330,1331,1333
Congenital nephrotic syndrome can be diagnosed from the foetal proteinuria and high levels of amniotic α-fetoprotein. Cystine storage disease can be diagnosed by the use of cultured fibroblasts from amniotic fluid.

256. **A B D** Ref:32,1331
Cysts in the liver do not cause any functional impairment. Surgical interference is required only for infection or major haemorrhage into a cyst.

257. **A D E** Ref:33,1353,1354,1355
In the earliest stages of acute obstruction dilatation of the urinary passages may be so small that it cannot be detected with ultrasound. An IVU may give useful information in total obstruction if it is performed before the affected kidney becomes non-functional.

258. **A D E** Ref:33,1357,1356
The urine will certainly be hypotonic and initial replacement therapy should be with half-normal saline. The diuresis may continue for several weeks.

259. **B D E** Ref:33,1371
Nephrotic syndrome and renal papillary necrosis have not been recorded. Outdated tetracycline can cause Fanconi's syndrome and penicillins can cause the acute nephritic syndrome.

260. **B C D** Ref:33,1375,1364,1376
Aspirin is more nephrotoxic than phenacetin or paracetamol, but taken alone it causes milder renal damage than combinations of analgesics such as aspirin-phenacetin-caffeine. Only some 20% of patients improve on withdrawal of analgesics: 50% remain stable and the remainder continue to deteriorate.

261. **A B** Ref:33,1362
Significant parenchymal damage may occur. The apparatus is complicated and expensive. Removal of fragments is necessary in 20-30% of cases.

262. **A B C E**   Ref:33,1344
Of patients with VUR when first seen, some 30% have established renal scarring.

263. **B C D E**   Ref:33,1346,1347
Nitrite testing is reliable in over 80% of patients.

264. **B**   Ref:33,1343,1342
VUR starts in infancy and has nearly always stopped by adolescence. Reflux nephropathy (the scarring acquired during childhood) is usually accompanied by stable renal function in adult life. Pregnancy presents special risks, including UTI, hypertension and the pre-eclamptic syndrome. The only indication for surgical correction is recurrent acute pyelonephritis not responding to medical treatment.

265. **A C D**   Ref:34,1380
Clubbing is not seen in B or E.

266. **A B D**   Ref:34,1414,1415
Chest signs include wide-spread crackles and wheezes and diminished breath-sounds at the bases. Controlled trials have not shown any benefit from prophylactic steroid therapy.

267. **A B C E**   Ref:34,1403,1404
Complications after trans-bronchial biopsy are uncommon with a combined rate for pneumothorax and minor haemoptysis of up to 9%.

268. **A B D E**   Ref:34,1393,1394,1396
TLC is raised in asthma. Carbon monoxide transfer may be increased in asthma owing to an increased exposure of capillary blood to the gas mixture.

269. **C D**   Ref:34,1407
The usual cells in A, B and E are lymphocytes.

270. **B C D**   Ref:34,1408
In histiocytosis, macrophage-like cells are seen containing X bodies; in pulmonary haemosiderosis, macrophages containing haemosiderin; in alveolar proteinosis, bilamellar material.

271. **C D**   Ref:34,1411
None of the cytotoxic drugs are free from the risk of causing

pulmonary damage; however this is a serious problem with bleomycin and to a lesser extent with busulphan. Cyclophosphamide and azathioprine rarely cause this trouble.

272.   **A B C D E**   **Ref:34,**1412
All are correct. Procainamide and hydralazine cause the 'drug-related lupus syndrome'.

273.   **A**   **Ref:35,**1421,1417,1419
The essential feature of chronic bronchitis is excessive production of bronchial mucus and Item A is its morphological counterpart. Items B, C and D are all characteristic of emphysema, not of bronchitis. Item E is found in the lungs of cigarette smokers and is thought to contribute to the development of centrilobular emphysema by the release of proteolytic enzymes.

274.   **A B D**   **Ref:35,**1424,1425
The PiZ phenotype is uncommon; patients having it are at high risk of developing panlobular emphysema in middle age. Patients with the PiMZ phenotype have a moderate reduction in serum antiprotease activity but have not been shown to be more susceptible to emphysema.

275.   **A C D**   **Ref:35,**1428
Tobacco and alcohol both increase hepatic theophylline metabolism.

276.   **A B D E**   **Ref:35,**1431
Filariasis may produce wheezing, with patchy opacities on X-ray, but does not interfere with the pulmonary circulation. *Schistosomiasis* involves passage of the parasites through the pulmonary vessels, sometimes causing blockage.

277.   **A C D E**   **Ref:35,**1433,1434
Therapy must continue for the rest of the patient's life.

278.   **A B E**   **Ref:35,**1436,1437
The responses to hypoxia and bronchopulmonary irritation are decreased.

279.   **B C D**   **Ref:35,**1448
In pulmonary infarction the effusion contains large numbers of

mesothelial cells, usually with erythrocytes. Mesothelioma produces malignant mesothelial cells.

280. **B C D E**   Ref:35,1450
A small pneumothorax (less than 20% of a hemithorax) may be treated on an out-patient basis. If more than 2 litres of air has been removed, an X-ray is necessary to check that the pneumothorax has been reduced; if not, there is probably a broncho-pleural fistula.

281. **A B E**   Ref:36,1470,1473,1474,1472
Some 20-40% of patients with small-cell cancer show a response to chemotherapy. There is no evidence that prophylactic cerebral irradiation prolongs survival.

282. **B D E**   Ref:36,1468,1469
Clubbing is commonest with squamous-cell carcinoma and is seen with some adenocarcinomas, but is rare with small-cell tumours.

283. **A B C**   Ref:36,1507,1508
Corticosteroids are ineffective, as are antibiotics; croup is a viral illness.

284. **B D**   Ref:36,1509,1510
The condition is caused by *Haemophilus influenzae*. There is no cough; a loud barking cough is characteristic of acute laryngo-tracheitis. Many strains of *H. influenzae* are resistant to ampicillin; the drug of choice is chloramphenicol.

285. **A B D E**   Ref:36,1494
Patients with a history of alcoholism or liver disease should only be treated in special circumstances.

286. **B E**   Ref:36,1506
Fever is usually present. Clinical signs in the chest are minimal. No technique for culture exists.

287. **A B E**   Ref:36,1485
SACE is not raised in fibrosing or allergic alveolitis.

288. **A C D**   Ref:36,1477,1478
Clubbing is seen in fewer than 10% of patients. Both chemotherapy and radiotherapy are uniformly ineffective.

289. **B D E**   Ref:37,1543,1545,1546
The level of eosinophilia in this case is higher than that usually seen in allergic bronchopulmonary aspergillosis. Pulmonary symptoms are unusual in ascariasis.

290. **A B C E**   Ref:37,1549,1548
Serum complement levels are normal.

291. **C D E**   Ref:37,1513,1514,1515,1516
The disease is extremely rare in Orientals. No lung disorder is present at birth; it is usually precipitated by a virus infection leading to secondary bacterial infection.

292. **A B D E**   Ref:37,1537
All may cause asthma except asbestos. Colophony is a resin used in the manufacturing of electronic devices.

293. **B C**   Ref:37,1552
There is no increased risk of tuberculosis or of lung cancer. Respirators are helpful but the mainstay of prevention is control of the dust level. The only treatment of the condition is that of the complications, e.g. infections and heart failure.

294. **A B E**   Ref:37,1555,1557
The WBC count is usually normal. Circulating rheumatoid and anti-nuclear factors are often present.

295. **B E**   Ref:37,1527,1528,1530
Skin allergy testing is rarely helpful. Non-specific avoidance of *possible* (rather than proven) allergens, e.g. by using special pillows and blankets, seldom produces much benefit.

296. **A C D E**   Ref:37,1519,1520
Goodpasture's syndrome involves a Type II reaction (cytotoxic) due to a reaction of specific antibodies with basement membranes of pulmonary alveoli (and of renal glomeruli).

297. **A C E**   Ref:38,1564,1565
Triglyceride release from lipid stores after trauma is increased by catecholamines and other factors and constitutes a major source of energy until the adipose tissue is exhausted. Hepatic protein synthesis increases greatly but this reflects production of 'acute phase' proteins

(complement, fibrinogen etc) at the expense of albumin, the synthesis of which *decreases*.

298.   B C D E   Ref:38,1562,1563,1565
Conversion of pyruvate to acetyl co-enzyme A is inhibited, the Krebs cycle is interrupted and lactate is produced (anaerobic glycolysis).

299.   C D   Ref:38,1582,1583,1585
No valid clinical distinction can be made between 'Gram-negative' septic shock and that due to Gram-positive bacteria, anaerobes, fungi, rickettsiae or viruses. The pulmonary vascular resistance is increased. The use of corticosteroids is controversial; some trials have shown benefit, others have not.

300.   A B C E   Ref:38,1569,1571
In most cases of diabetic ketoacidosis replacement with crystalloid solutions is perfectly adequate.

301   C E   Ref:38,1601,1602,1603
Expiration should be passive; negative pressure is nearly always unnecessary and may cause atelectasis. The I:E ratio should be 1:2. Some increase in inspired oxygen concentration is always desirable, to offset the disadvantages of assisted respiration.

302.   A B C E   Ref:38,1603
Sedation should be generous and may need to be combined with muscle relaxants.

303.   A C D   Ref:38,1593
ICP is reduced by hyperventilation which causes cerebral vasoconstriction. A fall in serum osmotic pressure leads to brain oedema and a rise in ICP; mannitol infusion has the opposite effects.

304.   B D E   Ref:38,1595,1596
It is now believed that all head injuries resulting in unconsciousness, however brief, cause structural damage, and the concept of 'concussion' is considered no longer tenable. Fatal brain damage can occur without any visible damage to scalp or skull.

305.   B C D   Ref:39,1621
See Figs. 3 and 4 of text.

306. A B D E Ref:39,1621
See Fig. 5 of text.

307. A B Ref:39,1637,1639,1638
The tumour lysis syndrome (following chemotherapy of bulky, highly sensitive tumours such as leukaemias and lymphomas) causes raised serum levels of potassium, inorganic phosphate and uric acid but *lowered* serum calcium. Treatment with cyclophosphamide in high doses may cause SIADH; the ectopic ACTH syndrome causes hypokalaemia.

308. A B D Ref:39,1635,1636
CT scanning shows evidence of meningeal involvement in about half of all patients. Irradiation of the affected area combined with intrathecal chemotherapy may give some palliation.

309. C D E Ref:39,1613,1614
CT scanning has little place in the diagnosis of primary growths of the gastrointestinal tract; barium studies and endoscopy are still the methods of choice. It can detect nodes involved by secondary growth when they are enlarged, but not before; involvement without enlargement is particularly a problem in pelvic cancer, where lymphography may demonstrate abnormal architecture in a normal-sized node.

310. A C Ref:39,1628,1629,1631
Megavoltage radiation is less absorbed by bone than orthovoltage radiation and the latter is often preferable when bony metastases are to be treated. Hair loss occurs in the area through which the radiation passes. Combined radio- and chemotherapy is often the preferred treatment.

311. C E Ref:39,1624
See Table 1 of text.

312. A B C Ref:39,1624
See Table 1 of text. The limiting side-effect for vincristine is neurotoxicity; and for bleomycin, lung damage.

313. A B C D Ref:40,1680
The relationship to oral contraception is not proven.

314.   **B D E**   Ref:**40,**1661,1662
Chemotherapy should in general be given first, as it gives some indication of response and may reduce the extent of surgery needed. Radio-isotope therapy is of no value in neuroblastoma; multiple chemotherapy or high-dose melphelan with bone-marrow transplantation offer the best hope.

315.   **B D E**   Ref:**40,**1669,1668,1670
The correct staging for item A is Stage II. Bone marrow involvement requires a marrow trephine for accurate diagnosis.

316.   **A B D E**   Ref:**40,**1666
Bone disease is not a feature.

317.   **A B D**   Ref:**40,**1654
The NAP score is low or zero; both serum B_{12} and serum B_{12} -binding protein are raised.

318.   **A C D**   Ref:**40,**1656
Chronic lymphocytic leukaemia is more common in men (2:1). Current therapy is not curative.

319.   **A C D E**   Ref:**40,**1657
The leukaemic cells arise from B-lymphocytes.

320.   **D E**   Ref:**40,**1685,1686
Most testicular tumours are painless when first seen; those which are painful may be misdiagnosed as epididymo-orchitis. Staging should be done *after* orchidectomy. The testis should be removed via an inguinal incision to avoid damage to the tunica albuginea.

321.   **A C**   Ref:**41,**1709,1710
Haemolysis is commonly both intra- and extravascular. The globin released in haemolysis is recycled for fresh haemoglobin production. The rate of urobilinogen excretion depends to some extent on microbial activity in the gut and is thus an unreliable indicator of the rate of haemolysis.

322.   **A B D**   Ref:**41,**1712,1713
The haemolytic crisis known as favism occurs when a G6PD-deficient person eats beans from the *Vicia fava* plant, i.e. broad beans, not

French beans (*Phaseolus vulgaris*). Penicillin does not cause haemolysis in G6PD deficiency.

323. **B D E**   Ref:41,1713
Inheritance is autosomal recessive. Onset is in childhood or even in the neo-natal period.

324. **C D E**   Ref:41,1718
Inheritance is autosomal dominant. The spherocytes are easily recognised in a standard blood smear. Splenectomy in early childhood carries a risk of subsequent pneumococcal or meningococcal septicaemia.

325. **B C D E**   Ref:41,1720,1721,1722
In nearly all patients with haemolytic anaemia due to IgG auto-antibodies, haemolysis is extravascular (liver or spleen).

326. **A B D E**   Ref:41,1695
Iron-binding capacity is usually reduced. A raised TIBC suggests iron deficiency.

327. **A C D E**   Ref:41,1696
The anaemia of chronic renal failure is normocytic or microcytic.

328. **A B D E**   Ref:41,1708,1707
The RBC folate level is reduced in more than 50% of cases of pernicious anaemia.

329. **A C D**   Ref:42,1753
See text.

330. **C E**   Ref:42,1757
Storage of blood causes losses principally of platelets and the labile coagulation factors (V and VIII); fibrinogen and the other coagulation factors are less affected.

331. **B C D E**   Ref:42,1740
The reaction is mediated by immunocompetent cells in the transfused blood.

332. **B E**   **Ref:42,1743,1744**
Platelet preparations inevitably contain some red cells and there is a
risk of immunising Rh-negative recipients. Patients with aplastic
anaemia should only be given platelets if they are bleeding;
prophylactic use will soon cause allo-immunisation. In DIC platelet
transfusion may be life-saving.

333. **B**   **Ref:42,1759**
Serial neutrophil counts provide no real warning of the onset; the
patient's symptoms (especially a sore throat) are the main guide. The
value of corticosteroids is unproven. Antibiotics are essential once
infection has developed. Leucocyte transfusions may be beneficial
when antibiotics fail.

334. **A B E**   **Ref:42,1759,1760**
Platelet transfusion may be beneficial when there is depression of
platelet production. Destruction of platelets by antibodies may be
reduced by corticosteroids.

335. **A D**   **Ref:42,1732,1733**
Females can be affected, either by the mating of a carrier with an
affected male, or by extreme 'Lyonisation' in a carrier. Severe
manifestations are only seen in those with 1% activity or less. The
prothrombin, thrombin clotting and bleeding times are all normal; the
activated partial thromboplastin time is prolonged.

336. **A C D**   **Ref:42,1736**
Many subjects in whom deficiency of von Willebrand's disease can be
demonstrated are asymptomatic. Presentation is usually with
bleeding from mucous membranes.

337. **A B E**   **Ref:43,1775**
Items C and D, although often found in schizophrenia, carry much
less diagnostic weight than the 'first-rank' symptoms (see Fig. 1 of
text).

338. **A D E**   **Ref:43,1776**
Prognosis is better with an acute onset and a known precipitating
cause.

339. A B   **Ref:43,1778**
ECT has no effect on delusions, hallucinations or other first-rank symptoms.

340. A B C D E   **Ref:43,1788**
All should be taken as indications of serious intent.

341. A B E   **Ref:43,1766,1767**
There is considerable interest in the possibility that 'slow' viruses may play a part, but so far no definite evidence. Aluminium intake has been suspected as an aetiological factor.

342. A B E   **Ref:43,1767,1768**
Dopaminergic drugs (e.g. amphetamine) make the positive symptoms worse. There is an increased incidence among those born in the *winter*.

343. A C D E   **Ref:43,1765**
Prostaglandins are not neuropeptides. See Fig. 3 of text.

344. B D   **Ref:43,1779,1785**
Sedatives and antidepressants are not usually needed. Stress-related conditions (e.g. ulcerative colitis) commonly become worse in bereavement. Occasionally grief progresses to severe depression and if this includes feelings of guilt or of being evil hospital admission should be considered.

345. A C D E   **Ref:44,1812**
The abdomen may be protuberant due to exaggerated lordosis but the navel is not effaced. The uterus may be enlarged up to the size of a 6-week pregnancy.

346. A C E   **Ref:44,1814**
The patient is psychiatrically normal at the time of delivery. Clinical findings may include acute schizophrenia with delusions and auditory hallucinations but much the commonest features are those of affective disorder, ranging through mania and hypomania to psychotic depression.

347. B D   **Ref:44,1800,1801**
The tablets should be taken in the evening so that the drowsiness induced combats insomnia. Amitriptyline and dothiepin cause

sedation; imipramine is non-sedating and protriptyline is stimulating. Overdose is highly toxic and in severe depression there is a risk of the drug being used in a suicidal attempt.

348. A B E   **Ref:44,**1809,1810
Only about 20% of cases of stupor are due to organic illness e.g. encephalitis, or lesions of brain-stem or third ventricle. In depressive stupor a single application of ECT can cause dramatic improvement lasting for hours or sometimes days.

349. A C   **Ref:44,**1831,1830,1832
Some 50% of children with recurrent pain continue to have symptoms when adult. Similar symptoms are often found in other members of the family. Treatment is normally by psychotherapy but marked anxiety may require the use of minor tranquillizers.

350. B E   **Ref:44,**1832
Control is expected by 4 years, not 3. The condition is more common in the USA than in Western Europe and is less common in upper social class.

351. A C E   **Ref:44,**1833
In night terrors there is total amnesia of the episode; the EEG shows arousal from slow-wave phase IV of sleep.

352. A B D   **Ref:44,**1833,1834
Boys are more often affected. Imipramine is effective.

353. B C D E   **Ref:45,**1860,1861
Benzodiazepines are not usually effective in controlling panic attacks; imipramine is probably the best drug.

354. B C D   **Ref:45,**1837
Hallucinations are commonly seen. Sedation may increase confusion and is best avoided if possible; in severe cases haloperidol is useful.

355. B D E   **Ref:45,**1846
Loss of 25% of original weight is required. Amenorrhoea occurs only when the weight loss is severe.

356. A B C D   **Ref:45,**1850
The parotid glands may be enlarged.

357. B E   **Ref:45,1850,1847**
Antidepressant drugs have been shown to be effective and should be used routinely. Group therapy is as effective as individual psychotherapy. The prognosis is better than for anorexia nervosa.

358. B C E   **Ref:46,1874**
Drugs of first choice would be A: carbamazepine, phenobarbitone, primidone or phenytoin; D: clonazepam or sodium valproate.

359. A C D E   **Ref:46,1875,1877**
Carbamazepine and phenobarbitone are enzyme inducers. Sodium valproate given in conjunction with phenobarbitone may cause severe sedation. Drug interactions with ethosuximide are rare.

360. A B C D   **Ref:46,1877**
Measurement of serum sodium valproate levels is only useful in detecting non-compliance and severe overdosage.

361. A D E   **Ref:46,1905,1904**
There is no familial incidence. The attacks come in clusters of one or more attacks (often at night) per 24 hours, for up to 6 weeks.

362. A B   **Ref:46,1884,1885**
Diazepam is absorbed in an unreliable fashion after IM injection; IV injection is best, or failing that rectal injection (not a suppository). Antibiotics should not be given until meningitis has been completely excluded. The EEG may help if the convulsion has been prolonged, focal, unilateral or repeated.

363. A B C E   **Ref:46,1886**
The sex of the child is immaterial.

364. A D E   **Ref:46,1888**
The figures for β and δ rhythms have been interchanged.

365. A B D   **Ref:46,1881**
Abductor pollicis brevis is supplied by the median nerve. Tibialis anterior is supplied by the peroneal branch of the sciatic nerve.

366. A C D   **Ref:47,1921,1922**
Hemiparesis, hemi-sensory loss, dysarthria and even hemianopia can occur in both carotid and vertebro-basilar ischaemia. However

amaurosis fugax and facial paresis are of unequivocal carotid origin;
dysphagia points conclusively to a vertebro-basilar event.

367. **A B C D E**   **Ref:47,**1924
All are legitimate indications for a CT scan; (A) to exclude
haemorrhage, (B) because the scan may confirm the diagnosis and
make lumbar puncture unnecessary, (C) because cerebellar
haematoma is treatable.

368. **A B E**   **Ref:47,**1935
The localising signs of cerebellar tumours (mid-line versus
hemisphere) have been transposed.

369. **A C D**   **Ref:47,**1938,1939
Glioblastoma multiforme is highly malignant and offers almost no
prospect of complete removal. Removal of cerebellar cystic
astrocytoma gives cure without recurrence in over 70% of cases.

370. **B**   **Ref:47,**1939,1938
Meningiomas are insensitive to radiotherapy and their correct
treatment and that of cerebellar cystic astrocytoma and of
haemangioblastoma, is radical removal whenever possible. Radiation
has little effect on glioblastomas.

371. **B E**   **Ref:47,**1930
The post-operative mortality is higher with early operation, probably
mainly due to cerebral ischaemia precipitated by the operation. There
is no convincing evidence of a lower overall mortality with early
operation.

372. **C D**   **Ref:47,**1953
Onset is usually between 30 and 50 years of age. Local neck pain is
common. Treatment with anticholinergic drugs, botulinum toxin or
surgical division of the appropriate nerves may be beneficial.

373. **B C E**   **Ref:47,**1912,1913
With an intact spinal cord some tendon reflexes may be retained. The
pupils must be fixed but need not be widely dilated.

374. **A D**   **Ref:47,**1947,1948
75% of patients with parkinsonism are underweight. Immobility may
lead to foot oedema. Impaired downward movement of the eyes

suggests progressive supranuclear palsy, which mimics the rigidity and hypokinesia of parkinsonism. Lack of blinking is a classical sign of parkinsonism.

375. **A C E**   **Ref:47,1916**
The condition is mainly seen in adults. Although the ventricles are enlarged, the pressure within them is not persistently raised and papilloedema is absent. However, CSF diversion sometimes leads to improvement.

376. **A C**   **Ref:48,1988,1989**
Muscle weakness is characteristically made worse by exercise, but is not associated with muscle pain. The tendon reflexes are generally brisk. Removal of a thymoma is advisable because of the risk of compression and infiltration of mediastinal structures, but there is usually no effect on the symptoms; however, in such patients immunosuppressive drugs are usually effective.

377. **B D**   **Ref:48,1992,1994**
Inheritance of DMD is X-linked; occurrence in a paternal relative would imply a new mutation in the propositus, an unlikely coincidence. Distribution of the myopathy is proximal and symmetrical. Pain and cramp suggest an inflammatory myopathy.

378. **A D**   **Ref:48,1995**
Death usually occurs between 20 and 30 years of age. The serum creatine kinase is only slightly raised. The carrier state can be identified by gene analysis in DMD and in dystrophia myotonica but not (at present) in Kugelberg-Welander disease.

379. **A C D E**   **Ref:48,2000**
The male/female ratio is 1.5 to 1. A myelogram is necessary to exclude a high cervical lesion.

380. **A C E**   **Ref:48,1973**
The principal root for triceps is C7 and for tibialis anterior L4.

381. **A C E**   **Ref:48,1977**
Pain may occur in the arm. The earliest sensory deficit is usually impairment of two-point discrimination.

382. **B E**   **Ref:48,1962**
Pain in the eyeball may precede visual loss by 1 or 2 days. The optic disc usually appears normal ('retrobulbar neuritis'). Improvement usually begins in 2 to 3 *weeks*.

383. **A D**   **Ref:48,1964,1965**
There is no consistent evidence of a persistent virus infection, though measles virus has been suspected. Auto-immunity to myelin basic protein, in experimental animals, produces allergic encephalitis but there is no evidence that this, or any other auto-immunity, plays a part in MS. No specific abnormality of lipid metabolism has so far been identified.

384. **A B D E**   **Ref:48,1958**
Hyperthyroidism may cause extreme agitation but not dementia; the latter can be caused by hypothyroidism. Thiamine deficiency is the basis of Korsakoff's syndrome.

385. **A C D**   **Ref:49,2009**
Involvement of the antecubital and popliteal fossae is characteristic in older children and adults.

386. **A D**   **Ref:49,2010**
The patients are usually adults. In coloured subjects the lesions are hyperpigmented. Corticosteroids should be given until the itching subsides.

387. **A B D**   **Ref:49,2004,2005**
Iron *deficiency* may cause generalised pruritus, as may polycythaemia vera.

388. **B C E**   **Ref:49,2041**
The lesions are usually solitary and occur usually on the hands, feet, glans penis or lips.

389. **C D E**   **Ref:49,2022,2024**
In general when the reaction is due to UV radiation alone, e.g. sunburn, polymorphous light eruption or solar urticaria, the shorter wavelength radiation, UVB (290-320 nm) is probably responsible. Where a sensitising mechanism is involved, as in C, D and E, the longer wavelengths (UVA) are more likely to be the cause.

390. A B C E   **Ref:49,2025**
Autoantibodies are found in A and C and in other associations with vitiligo (primary hyperthyroidism, hypothyroidism) and some autoimmune mechanism has been postulated but not proved. There is no association with acromegaly.

391. A B E   **Ref:49,2033**
Prognosis is worse in males and in the elderly.

392. A B   **Ref:49,2013,2015**
The pustules are sterile. Renal and hepatic damage may occur and the outcome may be fatal. A *short* course of prednisolone is sometimes beneficial, but long-term therapy makes the prognosis worse.

393. D   **Ref:50,2048,2049**
The condition is more common in women. Sunshine is an important precipitating factor, as is the incorrect use of topical corticosteroids. The condition is chronic and often persists for months or years if untreated.

394. A B D   **Ref:50,2055,2056**
Hirsutism is the growth of coarse terminal hair on women in a pattern similar to that seen in normal post-pubertal men; it is androgen-dependent. Hypertrichosis has a non-androgenic pattern and may be generalised or localised. Items C and E cause hair growth in the latter category, as do certain drugs eg. cyclosporin A, diazoxide and minoxidil.

395. C E   **Ref:50,2066,2065**
Ischaemic ulcers are usually on the lateral aspect of the leg, often higher than the malleolus. Surrounding pigmentation is characteristic of venous ulcers. Elastic support is contraindicated.

396. C D E   **Ref:50,2046,2047**
In a small minority of cases eating chocolate makes the condition worse; otherwise dietary control has no effect. Therapy in mild cases should begin with topical antimicrobial and keratolytic agents and systemic antibiotics should be given only when the topical agents produce no response.

397. **A B**   **Ref:50,2059,2057**
This condition is often known as 'common baldness'; it is dependent on the action of androgens (castrated males do not become bald). Item C describes the condition of 'telogen effluvium', a quite different entity. Some cases of androgenetic baldness in men respond to topical minoxidil. Cyproterone acetate is suitable for pre-menopausal women only.

398. **A B D**   **Ref:50,2071**
Some traces of chloasma may persist for many years. Telogen effluvium occurs post-partum and the scalp hair may not return to normal for over a year.

399. **B C D E**   **Ref:50,2062,2064**
Beau's lines are transverse grooves in the nails, separated by normal nail, due to recurrent illness. Arsenical poisoning produces *Mees' stripes* (transverse white bands on all nails).

400. **A D E**   **Ref:50,2069**
The eruption can occur in any area, including the face; the nodules are painful.

PLEASE NOTE

PasTest publications are available for the following postgraduate examinations:

MRCP Part 1 & 2	DCH
MRCGP	FRCS
MRCOG	FCAnaes Parts 1 & 2
DRCOG	PLAB

For details of the complete range of PasTest medical books and intensive revision courses please write for a copy of our catalogue which will be sent to you by return of post.

**PasTest, Egerton Court, Parkgate Estate,
Knutsford, Cheshire WA16 8DX**